# PREP

### PROGRAM REVIEW & EXAM PREPARATION

# DENTAL ASSISTANT

**Emily Andujo, RDH, BS, MS**
Dental Hygiene Education
Pima Community College
Tucson, Arizona

APPLETON & LANGE
Stamford, Connecticut

Copyright © 1997 by Appleton & Lange
A Simon & Schuster Company

97 98 99 00 01 / 10 9 8 7 6 5 4 3 2 1

Prentice Hall International (UK) Limited, *London*
Prentice Hall of Australia Pty. Limited, *Sydney*
Prentice Hall Canada, Inc., *Toronto*
Prentice Hall Hispanoamericana, S.A., *Mexico*
Prentice Hall of India Private Limited, *New Delhi*
Prentice Hall of Japan, Inc., *Tokyo*
Simon and Schuster Asia Pte. Ltd., *Singapore*
Editora Prentice Hall do Brasil Ltda., *Rio de Janeiro*
Prentice Hall, *Upper Saddle River, New Jersey*

**Library of Congress Cataloging-in-Publication Data**

Dental assistant : PREP : program review & exam preparation / [edited
  by] Emily Andujo. — 1st ed.
       p.    cm.
    Rev. ed. of: Appleton & Lange's review for the dental assistant.
  3rd ed. / Emily Andujo. c1992.
    Includes bibliographical references and index.
    ISBN 0-8385-1513-4 (alk. paper)
    1. Dental assistants—Examinations, questions, etc.  2. Dentistry—
  Examinations, questions, etc.  I. Andujo, Emily.  II. Andujo,
  Emily   Appleton & Lange's review for the dental assistant.
  III. Appleton & Lange's review for the dental assistant.
    [DNLM:  1. Dental Care—examination questions.  2. Dental
  Assistants—examination questions.    WU 18.5 D413 1997]
  RK60.5.H57    1997
  617.6'01'076—dc20
  DNLM/DLC
  for Library of Congress                              96-9709
                                                         CIP

Acquisitions Editor: Marinita Timban
Production Editor: Elizabeth Ryan
Designer: Libby Schmitz

PRINTED IN THE UNITED STATES OF AMERICA

0-8385-1513-4

9 780838 515136

90000

*This book is dedicated
to all dental assistants and
dental assisting students who aspire to
excel in their chosen profession*

# Contents

# Contributors

**Stephanie Dante, CDA, RDA, AS**
Instructor, Dental Practice Management
Department of Dental Assisting
Cerritos Community College
Norwalk, California
*Dental Management*

**Joleen Failor, CDA, RDA, BVE**
Director, Department of Dental Assisting
Division of Health Occupations
Cerritos Community College
Norwalk, California
*Chairside Assisting*

**Robert Hankel, DDS**
Dental Management Consultant
Dental Practice Broker
Adjunct Faculty
Pima Community College
Tucson, Arizona
*Dental Management*

**Adelle Krayer, RDH, BA, MA**
Assistant Professor
Dental Hygiene Department
Cerritos College
Lecturer, University California Los Angeles
Infection Control & OSHA Compliance Consultant
*Infection Control*
*Occupational Safety*

**Richard J. Nagy, DDS, BA**
Director, Department of Periodontics
Veterans Administration Medical Center
    West Los Angeles
Lecturer, University of California, Los Angeles,
    School of Dentistry
Los Angeles, California
Staff Dentist
Rancho Los Amigos Hospital
Downey, California
*Biomedical Sciences—Oral Pathology*
*Medical Emergencies*

**Joan Otomo-Corgel, DDS, MPH**
Adjunct Assistant Professor
Department of Periodontics
University of California, Los Angeles,
    School of Dentistry
Los Angeles, California
Faculty, Staff Dentist
Veterans Administration
Medical Center
    West Los Angeles
Staff Dentist
Rancho Los Amigos Hospital
Downey, California
*Preventive Dentistry*
*Biomedical Sciences—Pharmacology, Oral Pathology*
*Chairside Assisting—Periodontics*

**Virginia F. Santos, CDA, RDA, BVE**
Director, Department of Dental Assisting (Retired)
Division of Health Science
East Los Angeles Occupational Center
Los Angeles, California
*Chairside Assisting—Orthodontics*

**Jane M. Watanabe, CDA, RDA, OSMA, MSEd**
Administrative Coordinator, Oral and
    Maxillofacial Surgery
Surgical Assistant for Implant Program
Former Coordinator Department
    of Auxiliary Utilization
University of Southern California
    School of Dentistry
Los Angeles, California
*Chairside Assisting—Oral and
    Maxillofacial Surgery*

**Donna J. Wedell, CDA, RDA, AS**
Instructor, Radiology and Dental Science
Department of Dental Assisting
Cerritos Community College
Norwalk, California
*Dental Radiology*

**Sheila D. Whetstone, RDH, BHS**
Medical Education Program Coordinator
Veterans Administration Medical Center
Long Beach, California
*Dental Radiology*

**Rizkalla Zakhary, PhD**
Associate Professor of Anatomy (Retired)
Department of Basic Sciences
University of Southern California
   School of Dentistry
Los Angeles, California
*General Anatomy*
*Dental Anatomy*

*In Memoriam*
*Bernice Hart, CDA, and Jackie Crager, CDA*
*For their exemplary dedication and commitment to*
*maintaining the highest standards of the dental*
*assisting profession and to their devotion to*
*dental assisting education.*

# Preface

*Dental Assistant: Program Review and Exam Preparation (PREP)* serves as an adjunct to regular dental science course work, extracting fundamental key concepts from reading assignments and class notes. This review book has been prepared to help students and dental assistants direct their study efforts towards exam-related material, particularly the Dental Assistant National Board Certification Examinations.

*Dental Assistant: PREP* is divided into ten chapters and provides a detailed overview of the topics addressed in each of the six dental assisting certification examinations: General Chairside Examination, Infection Control Examination, Dental Radiation Health and Safety Examination, Orthodontic Assisting Examination, Oral and Maxillofacial Surgery Assisting Examination, and the Dental Practice Management Assisting Examination. The content of the material presented in each of the ten chapters is focused on exam-related material directing the outline of study and exam preparation for the test candidate. Additional examination preparation material is provided in the companion book, *Appleton & Lange's Quick Review: Dental Assistant,* which contains 1000 sample test questions written in the format of the six certification examinations. Both books provide a thorough preparation for the certification examinations administered by the Dental Assisting National Board (DANB).

## KEY FEATURES AND USE

- A **list of key terms** at the start of each section identifies important terms or phrases essential for the student to know. The student will find it helpful to write the definition of each term before beginning each section.
- **Illustrations** are used to appeal to the visual learner as well as the verbal learner and enhance understanding of the subject matter.
- The **summary boxes** serve to call the student's attention to the most important facts in a particular section. Students can use summary boxes as an overview of key information.
- A **glossary** of frequently used terms and abbreviations associated with the Infection Control Certification Examination is included to provide students with a resource tool for understanding the terminology used in the study of infection control and occupational safety.
- The **Review Questions** allow students to assess chapter material. Exact page references follow each question, providing answers in chapter material. Following completion of the chapter review questions the student is ready for final self-

evaluation by answering sample test questions in the companion book, *Appleton & Lange's Quick Review: Dental Assistant*.

# SPECIFIC INFORMATION ABOUT THE CERTIFICATION EXAMINATION

The official source of all information with respect to the Dental Assistant Certification Examination is the Dental Assisting National Board (DANB), 216 E. Ontario Street, Chicago, IL 60611. Qualification for certification must be met before sitting for the examination. Several eligibility pathways are defined by the certifying board, and the candidate must submit written proof of eligibility directly to the DANB. A formal application must be completed before the appropriate deadline and accompanied by the required fee in order to sit for the certification examination.

Approximate examination testing time is 4 hours and 15 minutes. Test results will require approximately 6 to 8 weeks from the date of testing to be processed and mailed. Examination results are not released by phone.

If taking only the Infection Control or Radiation Health and Safety Examination, testing time will be 1 hour and 15 minutes. If taking the General Chairside Examination only, testing time will be 1 hour and 45 minutes. If taking the Orthodontic or Oral and Maxillofacial Surgery Assisting Examinations only, testing time will be 2 hours and 45 minutes.

## *EXAMINATION QUESTION FORMATS*

The certification examination includes four different question formats: *one best answer—single item, complex multiple choice* or *K-type, negative format,* and *matching*. In some cases, a group of questions may be related to a dental charting exercise or dental condition for interpretation. Some of the items are stated in the negative. In such instances, the negative word is in capital letters (eg, "All of the following are correct EXCEPT," "Which of the following choices is NOT correct?" *and* "Which of the following is LEAST correct?"). Additionally, some questions have illustrative material (instruments, x-rays, tables) that will require further understanding and interpretation on your part.

**One Best Answer—Single Item Question.** This type of question presents a problem or asks a question and is followed by four choices, only one of which is entirely correct. The directions preceding this type of question generally will appear as follows.

**DIRECTIONS (Question 1): Each of the questions or incomplete statements in this section is followed by four suggested answers or completions. Select the ONE lettered answer or completion that is BEST in each case.**

An example of this item type follows.

1. The most important reason for using alginate for preliminary impressions is the
   A. pleasant color and taste of the material
   B. speed and simplicity of mixing
   C. ability of alginate to withstand the pouring of multiple models from a single impression
   D. greater precision of alginate as compared to hydrocolloid

   In this type of question, choices other than the correct answer may be partially correct, but there can only be one best answer. In Question 1, the key word is "most." Although alginate impression material is pleasant tasting, has a pleasing color, and is easy to mix, these factors do not account for using alginate impressions material for preliminary impression procedures. Hydrocolloid impression material is used for final impression procedures only and is not used to take preliminary working impressions. Thus, the most important reason can only be (C) ability of alginate to withstand the pouring of multiple models from a single impression.

**Complex Multiple Choice—K-type Question.** These questions are considered the most difficult and you should be certain that you understand and follow the code that always accompanies these questions:

**DIRECTIONS (Question 2): For each of the items in this section, ONE or MORE of the numbered options is correct. Choose answer**
   A. **if only 1, 2, and 3 are correct**
   B. **if only 1 and 3 are correct**
   C. **if only 2 and 4 are correct**
   D. **if only 4 is correct**
   E. **if all are correct**

   This code is always the same (i.e., D would never say "if 3 is correct"), and it is repeated throughout the exam whenever there are multiple complex—K-type item questions.
   A sample question follows:

2. Some benefits of tray setups are
   1. they save time setting up
   2. the dentist sets them up for the assistant
   3. they eliminate delay in searching for instruments
   4. they are used only in restorative procedures

---

**BOX 1. STRATEGIES FOR ANSWERING ONE BEST ANSWER—SINGLE ITEM QUESTIONS**

- Remember that only one choice can be the correct answer.
- Read the question carefully to be sure that you understand what is being asked.
- Quickly read each choice for familiarity. (This important step is often not done by test takers.)
- Go back and consider each choice individually.
- If a choice is partially correct, tentatively consider it to be incorrect. (This step will help you lessen your choices and increase your odds of choosing the correct answer.)
- Consider the remaining choices and select the one you think is the answer. At this point, you may want to quickly scan the stem to be sure you understand the question and your answer.
- Fill in the appropriate circle on the answer sheet. (Even if you do not know the answer, you should use your best judgment and make a selection. You are scored on the number of correct answers, so **do not leave any blanks**.)

**BOX 2. STRATEGIES FOR ANSWERING COMPLEX MULTIPLE CHOICE— K-TYPE QUESTIONS**

- Carefully read and become familiar with the accompanying directions to this tricky question type.
- Read the stem to be certain that you know what is being asked.
- Read through each of the numbered choices. If you can determine whether any of the choices is true or false, you may find it helpful to place a "+" (true) or a "–" (false) next to the number.
- Focus on the numbered choices and your true/false notations, and use the following sequence to logically determine the correct answer.
1. Note that in the answer code choices 1 and 3 are *always* both either true or false together. If you are sure that either one is incorrect, your answer must be (C) or (D).
2. If you are sure that choice 2 and either choice 2 *or* 3 are incorrect, your answer must be (D).
3. If you are sure that choices 2 and 4 are incorrect, your answer must be (B).
- Only one circle on the answer sheet must be filled in.

You first need to determine which choices are right and wrong and then which code corresponds to the correct numbers. In question 2, statements 1 and 3 are true, and therefore (B) is the correct answer.

**Negative Format Question.** This type of question is used to test the exception to a general rule or principle. These questions can be tricky, since they require a reverse logic of reasoning for the examinee.

**DIRECTIONS (Question 3): Each of the items or incomplete statements in this section is followed by suggested answers or completions. Select the ONE lettered answer or completion that is the EXCEPTION or false statement.**

An example of this item type follows.

3. All of the following statements apply to interdental brushes EXCEPT
    A. they are useful in removing interproximal plaque
    B. they are used where there is a space between the teeth
    C. they are useful even when it is possible to remove plaque with a toothbrush around healthy tissues
    D. they are useful in exposed furcation areas

Note that unlike the one best answer—single item question style, the negative format question is asking you to select the one answer that is false or the exception. Carefully read each of the choices to determine the positive options first. Remember that positive choices can be safely eliminated, since you are being asked to select the choice that is false. This process of elimination is sometimes easier to think through and allows the correct choice—the exception—to stand out quickly. In this particular case, option choices (A), (B), and (D) are positive or true in reference to interdental brushes and are, therefore, incorrect answer choices. By eliminating these three positive options, only choice (C) remains. Choice (C) is the correct answer because it is the exception, or false statement. If plaque can be removed easily with a toothbrush and the tissue is healthy, an interdental brush is not necessary.

**Matching Question.** These questions are essentially matching questions that are always accompanied by the following general directions.

**DIRECTIONS (Questions 4 through 8): Match the items in Column A with their primary function in Column B.**

A sample matching series follows.

**BOX 3. STRATEGIES FOR ANSWERING NEGATIVE FORMAT QUESTIONS**

- Remember that you are using reverse logic reasoning.
- Focus on words that are capitalized in the stem of the question.
- Consider each choice option individually. Note that the incorrect options of a negative format question are written in a positive form.
- Your circled answer is the option choice that is the exception or least correct.

COLUMN A
4. spoon excavator
5. condenser
6. scaler
7. discoid–cleoid
8. ball burnisher

COLUMN B
A. used to pack filling material
B. finishes or smooths restorations
C. effective in excavating soft caries
D. used for removal of cement
E. refines occlusal anatomy

A series of five questions usually is listed under Column A, with five answer choices under Column B. In this particular matching set, dental instruments are listed under Column A. Select the first item, question 4, spoon excavator, and systematically proceed to Column B, carefully reading all of the options and considering each choice individually. Continue this process with each item question 5, 6, 7, and 8. After reading each possible option in Column B, determine your correct choice on the answer sheet. As with single item questions, only one choice can be correct for a given question. For this reason, it is best to run through each question with all five option choices before entering your final answers. The correct answers for the matching set are as follows: 4 (C), 5 (A), 6 (D), 7 (E), 8 (B).

## EXAMINATION SCORING

Because there is no deduction for wrong answers, you should answer every question. The certification examination is not graded on a curve. Your test is scored in the following way.

1. The Certified Dental Assisting Examination consists of a total of 320 test questions; 120 questions are derived from general chairside assisting subject matter, 100 questions are derived from radiation health and safety, and 100 questions are derived from infection control. The test candidate must answer a minimum number of questions correctly in each of these three subject areas in order to successfully pass the certification examination. These minimum passing standards are calculated according to the number of correctly answered questions, which are individually scored according to item subject matter content and value of importance.

2. The Specialty Certification Examination in Dental Practice Management consists of a total of 275 test questions; 275 questions are specifically derived from that particular dental specialty.

   The Specialty Certification Examination in Oral and Maxillofacial Surgery consists of a total of 320 test questions; 220 questions are derived specifically from that particular dental specialty and the remaining 100 questions are derived from infection control.

   The Specialty Certification Examination in Orthodontics consists of a total of 300 questions; 200 questions are derived specifically from that particular dental specialty and the remaining 100 questions are derived from infection control. The test candidate must answer a minimum number of questions based on each of these sections correctly in order to successfully pass the specialty certification examinations.

The examination may be repeated if failed following guidelines established by the DANB. Examination results are released in writing and issued directly to the test candidate only. All test candidates who pass the certification examinations successfully will receive a certificate designating them as a Certified Dental Assistant or a credential certifying them in a particular dental assisting specialty.

## PHYSICAL CONDITIONS

The DANB is very concerned that all their examinations be administered under uniform conditions in the numerous centers that are used. All test candidates are advised to protect the integrity of their answer choices. If the test candidate feels that the testing site facilities are too crowded or arranged in such a manner that would make it difficult to protect the answers, the candidate should inform the testing site test administrator immediately.

Except for a No. 2 pencil and eraser, you are not permitted to bring anything (books, notes, reference materials) into the test room. A calculator is permitted for the Dental Practice Management Specialty Examination only. All candidates are required to bring their assigned admission card on the day of the examination and appropriate identification. No questions concerning the content matter of the examination may be asked during the testing session. Furthermore, no visitors will be permitted during the examination session. Late comers may be admitted but will not be allowed to write beyond the allotted examination testing time period.

# Acknowledgments

My sincere appreciation and thanks is expressed to Marinita Timban, Review Book Editor at Appleton & Lange for her support and cooperation with the Dental Assistant review for the PREP Series. Additional thanks is extended to Amy Schermerhorn, Editorial Associate, for her continued assistance with this project.

I would also like to thank my friends, colleagues, and contributors for their suggestions and encouragement. In particular to Olivia Ordonez, CDA, Dental Office Manager & Safety Coordinator for her assistance and contribution to the chapter on Occupational Safety and to Lori Gagliardi, RDA, RDH, for her input on the content.

Major credit for art work and coordination of illustrations goes to Arthur V. Dorame, Medical Illustrator, VA Medical Center, West Los Angeles, and to Terry G. Hudson, CDT, VA Dental Service, for his technical expertise and invaluable contributions to the chapter on Dental Radiology.

A special note of thanks to my computer mentor and soul mate for the extra patience displayed and the countless hours spent formatting, inputting, and editing this project to final perfection for copy. Thanks, "D."

# Biomedical Sciences

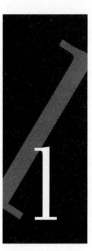

## I. INTRODUCTION

In order to provide appropriate patient treatment and care, a fundamental knowledge of the interrelationship between general health and oral health is necessary. To understand this relationship, the dental auxiliary must have a firm foundation in the basic health sciences, including anatomy and physiology (Table 1–1). This chapter provides an overview of the major systems of the human body, their physiologic functions, and significance to dental health. A synopsis of the closely related biomedical sciences of microbiology, oral pathology, and pharmacology is also presented.

TABLE 1–1. SYSTEMS OF THE BODY

| | |
|---|---|
| 1. Skeletal system | 6. Respiratory system |
| 2. Muscular system | 7. Digestive system |
| 3. Nervous system | 8. Excretory system |
| 4. Circulatory system | 9. Endocrine system |
| 5. Lymphatic system | 10. Reproductive system |

## II. SYSTEMS OF THE BODY

### Key Terms ◀

| | | |
|---|---|---|
| *ARTERY* | *BONE MARROW* | *DIGESTION* |
| *ARTICULATION* | *CRANIAL NERVES* | *HOMEOSTASIS* |
| *AXIAL* | *DETOXIFICATION* | *HORMONES* |

*LYMPHADENOPATHY*          *PLATELETS*          *SALIVA*

*LYMPHOCYTES*              *PTYALIN*            *SYMPATHETIC*

*PARASYMPATHETIC*          *RESPIRATION*        *VEINS*

---

## A.   SKELETAL SYSTEM

Bone is a rigid form of connective tissue that contains cells in an intercellular matrix or ground substance. Three types of cells are associated with bone: osteoblasts, osteocytes, and osteoclasts. Osteoblasts are involved with bone formation and are found near those surfaces of bones where the intercellular matrix is deposited. Osteocytes, or matrix bone cells, are osteoblasts that have become trapped within the intercellular matrix. Osteoclasts are giant cells that possess many nuclei and are responsible for the breakdown of bone. Bone contains a substance known as **bone marrow.** The function of the bone marrow is the production of red blood cells, white blood cells, and platelets, which are the main components of blood.

| Cells of Bones |
| --- |
| Osteoblasts<br>Osteocytes<br>Osteoclasts<br>Bone marrow |

The main functions of bone are support and protection. The skeleton, which consists of 206 bones, provides support for the body and enables a human to stand in an erect position. The bones protect many vital organs, provide locations for muscle attachments, and store minerals.

The skeleton is divided into two parts: axial and appendicular. The **axial** skeleton is comprised of the skull, vertebral column, and ribcage. The appendicular skeleton is comprised of bones associated with the body's appendages.

| Skeletal System |
| --- |
| Axial skeleton<br>Skull<br>Vertebral column<br>Ribcage<br>Appendicular skeleton<br>Bones of the body's appendages |

Bones are connected at joints or **articulations.** There are three types of joints: synarthrotic, amphiarthrotic, and diarthrotic. Synarthrotic joints join bones in close contact and do not move. Examples include the sutures, which are the joints between the bones in the skull. Amphiarthrotic joints have limited movement. Diarthrotic joints are freely movable and are the most common joints found in the body. Examples include the elbow, knee, and wrist. The temporomandibular joint, joining the maxilla and mandible, is a diarthrotic joint.

| Basic Types of Joints |
| --- |
| Synarthrotic joints—suture type<br>Amphiarthrotic joints—limited<br>   movement<br>Diarthrotic joints—freely movable |

## B.   MUSCULAR SYSTEM

Muscle cells or fibers are grouped into bundles that are responsible for producing movement. Muscle fibers require a rich blood supply to work effectively. These blood vessels, as well as nerves, are carried in connective tissue, which also serves to bind the muscle fibers together. There are three types of muscle: striated, smooth, and cardiac.

| Types of Muscle |
| --- |
| Striated<br>Smooth<br>Cardiac |

Striated muscle is found attached to the skeleton and is voluntary in its action. Striated muscle has a microscopic appearance of numerous cross-striations. Smooth muscles, also known as involuntary muscles, are not consciously controlled and are located within the wall structures of the organ systems, such as the digestive and respiratory systems.

Cardiac muscle is specialized muscle found in the heart. It is an involuntary muscle that is responsible for contraction of the heart and circulation of blood.

Muscle reflexes are actions causing an uncontrollable reaction, such as gagging, swallowing, and coughing.

## C. NERVOUS SYSTEM

Nervous tissue is distributed widely throughout the body. The nervous system consists of those tissues that collect stimuli from the environment, transform the stimuli into impulses, and transmit these impulses to highly organized receptor areas, where they are interpreted, and the appropriate response is made.

There are two major segments of the nervous system: the central nervous system, composed of the brain and the spinal cord, and the peripheral nervous system, composed of all other nerves of the body.

The **cranial nerves** are 12 paired nerves that control many major functions of the body, including sight, smell, and taste (Table 1–2).

Also included in the peripheral nervous system is the autonomic nervous system, composed of neurons that innervate internal organs and perform such basic life functions as digestion, respiration, and regulation of the heart. The autonomic nervous system is responsible for maintaining bodily **homeostasis** (equilibrium and physiologic stability) and is subdivided into the **sympathetic** and **parasympathetic** nervous systems.

When stimulated, the sympathetic nervous system accelerates the heart beat, produces thick, viscous saliva, and decreases motility and tone of the gastrointestinal tract. Conversely, when the parasympathetic nervous system is stimulated, the heart beat is slowed, watery saliva is produced, and motility and tone of the gastrointestinal system are increased. Although these two parts of the autonomic nervous system appear to be antagonistic in nature, their dual action maintains homeostasis.

The nervous system is perhaps one of the most important systems related to dentistry, since stimuli, such as pain and anxiety, of-

### Components of Nervous System

Central Nervous System
  • Brain and spinal cord
Peripheral Nervous System
  • Autonomic
  • Sympathetic
  • Parasympathetic

TABLE 1–2.  CRANIAL NERVES

| CRANIAL NERVES | FUNCTION |
|---|---|
| I   Olfactory | Smell |
| II   Optic | Sight |
| III   Oculomotor | Movement of eyes |
| IV   Trochlear | Movement of eyes |
| V   Trigeminal | Chewing, conduction of sensation, and movement by the ophthalmic, maxillary, and mandibular nerves to the face |
| VI   Abducens | Movement of eyes |
| VII   Facial | Secretion of saliva, taste, facial expression |
| VIII   Auditory (acoustic) | Hearing and balance |
| IX   Glossopharyngeal | Taste, swallowing, secretion of saliva |
| X   Vagus | Slowing of heart beat, increase in peristaltic movement |
| XI   (Spinal) Accessory | Movement of shoulder and head |
| XII   Hypoglossal | Movement of tongue, speech |

ten occur. Nerve fibers are ubiquitous in the oral cavity. Therefore, any deviation from the norm usually results in an unpleasant situation. The use of anesthesia to block the sensation of pain is of primary importance. A local anesthetic prevents a nerve fiber from firing when a stimulus is applied.

Paresthesia, a sensation of anesthesia caused by nerve damage, can result from trauma to a nerve during the administration of anesthesia or from the surgical removal of a tooth. It can be temporary or permanent.

Trigeminal neuralgia is a nerve disturbance involving the oral cavity and face. The etiologic factors are varied, but the clinical effect is searing or stabbing facial pain. This condition can be temporary or permanent.

Common diseases associated with the nervous system include Parkinson's disease, epilepsy, and Bell's palsy (paralysis of the facial nerve).

## Summary

- The human skeleton consists of 206 bones and is divided into two parts, axial and appendicular.
- Within bone is a substance known as bone marrow which produces red blood cells, white blood cells, and platelets.
- Bones are connected at joints or articulations. Synarthrotic joints do not move and join bones in close contact—examples include the joints (sutures) of the bones of the skull.
- The temporomandibular joint is an example of a diarthrotic joint.
- There are three types of muscle: striated, smooth, and cardiac.
- Muscle reflexes are actions causing an uncontrollable reaction such as gagging, swallowing, and coughing.
- The nervous system is composed of the central nervous system (brain and spinal cord) and the peripheral nervous system.
- The cranial nerves control major functions of the body including sight, smell, and taste.
- The autonomic nervous system is responsible for maintaining bodily homeostasis (equilibrium and physiologic stability) and is subdivided into the sympathetic and parasympathetic nervous systems.

## D.   CIRCULATORY SYSTEM

The circulatory system is comprised of the heart, blood vessels, and blood. The heart is a specialized organ of the body responsible for initiating the flow of the blood through the body. It is a pump composed of four chambers: left and right atria and left and right ventricles.

After blood leaves the heart, it travels through the arteries, capillaries, and veins. **Arteries** carry blood away from the heart to all other parts of the body. They are relatively thick, elastic vessels that expand and contract as the heart pumps blood. The pulse rate is the number of heart contractions during a given period of time. When the heart contracts, systole occurs. When the heart is in a relaxed phase, diastole occurs. The measurement of arterial pressure generated during systole and diastole corresponds to the body's blood pressure. For example, the average normal pressure is 120/80, measured in millimeters of mercury (mm Hg), which means 120 systole and 80 diastole.

**Veins** carry blood back to the heart, are thinner than arteries, ◀
and possess small valves that prevent blood from flowing back-
ward. Unlike the blood flow in arteries, the blood in veins flows
smoothly.

Capillaries are the smallest blood vessels and appear in the
greatest number. It is at the capillary level that the blood and cells
exchange nutrients, oxygen, and waste products.

**1.    Blood.** Each adult has 10 to 12 pints (4.7 to 5.6 liters) of blood.
Blood is composed of a liquid component called plasma and of solid
components that include red blood cells, white blood cells, and
platelets.

Plasma is 90% water. The remaining 10% is divided among
plasma proteins (globulin and fibrinogen), inorganic salts, and other
products (hormones, antibodies, urea, oxygen, carbon dioxide, and
products of digestion). Globulin functions in the body's defense system, and fibrinogen is an integral component in the clotting of
blood.

**2.    Red Blood Cells.** The solid constituents of blood include the red
blood cells, white blood cells, and platelets. Red blood cells, or erythrocytes, are donut-shaped discs that have no nuclei. They are produced in bone marrow and contain hemoglobin, an iron-containing
protein responsible for transporting oxygen to the cells.

**3.    White Blood Cells.** White blood cells, or leukocytes, are larger
than red blood cells and include neutrophils, basophils, and lymphocytes. Some white blood cells are formed in bone marrow and some
in the lymphatic system. Neutrophils are the most common type of
white blood cells. They are phagocytes (cell eaters), which function
in areas of inflammation by ingesting foreign debris. Basophils are
the second most common white blood cells, and function in the production of the anticoagulant heparin. **Lymphocytes** are an integral ◀
part of the body's defense mechanisms.

**4.    Platelets. Platelets,** which play a critical role in the clotting pro- ◀
cess, are actually fragments of larger cells called megakaryocytes,
which are formed in bone marrow.

Blood type is inherited and remains unchanged throughout life.
There are four basic blood types: A, B, AB, and O. These categories
are based on the presence of certain antibodies and the degree to
which the red blood cells agglutinate (clump together). In addition,
blood types are subdivided by the presence or absence of certain
groups of proteins or antigens.

| Circulatory System |
| --- |
| Heart |
| Blood vessels |
| Blood |
| Red blood cells—erythrocytes |
| White blood cells—leukocytes |
| Platelets |

## Summary

- The circulatory system is comprised of the heart, blood vessels,
  and the blood.
- Arteries carry blood away from the heart to all other parts of the
  body.
- Veins carry blood back to the heart.
- The measurement of arterial pressure generated during systole
  and diastole corresponds to the body's blood pressure.
- Blood and cells exchange nutrients, oxygen, and waste products
  at the capillary level.

- Blood is composed of red blood cells (erythrocytes) which contain hemoglobin, an iron containing protein responsible for transporting oxygen to the cells.
- White blood cells, or leukocytes, are larger than red blood cells and include neutrophils, basophils, and lymphocytes. White blood cells play an integral role in the body's defense mechanisms.
- Platelets are formed in the bone marrow and play a critical role in the clotting process.

## E.  LYMPHATIC SYSTEM

The lymphatic system works in close association with the circulatory system. The purpose of the lymphatic system is to return intercellular fluid and materials to the circulatory system. The fluid and returning materials are called lymph. The lymphatic system also serves to transport absorbed fats from the intestines to the blood and plays an integral part in the body's defense systems.

The organs of the lymphatic system include lymph nodes, tonsils, the thymus, and the spleen. Lymph nodes are encapsulated masses of lymph tissue that filter the lymph fluid and produce lymphocytes and monocytes, which destroy micoorganisms in the body. The tonsils and the thymus serve in similar capacities, although their function is still not completely understood. The spleen acts as a storage area for red blood cells and has other important functions.

If larger amounts of tissue fluid collect in an area because of a blockage in the lymphatic system or a change in the protein concentration of the surrounding intercellular fluid, a pathologic state called edema results. Edema is often symptomatic of other bodily pathologies, a reaction to a localized inflammatory process, or both.

▶    **Lymphadenopathy,** or swelling of the lymph nodes, should alert the dentist and dental assistant to an infectious process in the patient's body (Fig. 1–1).

---

### Lymphatic System Organs

Lymph nodes
Tonsils
Thymus
Spleen

---

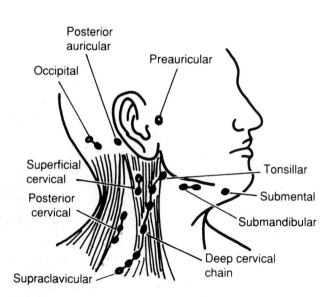

Figure 1–1.  Lymph nodes of the head and neck.

## F.   RESPIRATORY SYSTEM

**Respiration** is the process whereby the oxygen required by each ◀
cell for the production of energy is introduced into the bloodstream,
and carbon dioxide, a waste product of cellular activity, is removed.
This transfer of gases occurs in the lungs where thin-walled capillaries are in close proximity to the alveoli, or air sacs, of the lungs. Air
is inhaled through the nose and enters the nasal sinuses, where it is
filtered, warmed, and moistened. The air then travels through the na-
sopharynx to the pharynx, and past the glottis, which is the opening
into the larynx and trachea. The epiglottis is a protective flap of tissue that prevents food from entering the lungs. After passing through
the glottis, air enters the larynx and subsequently enters the trachea,
the major duct leading to the lungs. The trachea branches out into
smaller ducts called bronchi, which in turn divide into bronchioles
and finally alveoli, the smallest components of the respiratory system.

Air is inspired by expansion of the ribcage and diaphragm,
causing a negative air pressure against the lungs. The lungs expand
as air is drawn into them.

After the exchange of gases, air pressure around the lungs increases while the diaphragm and ribcage relax. As the air pressure
increases, the air is forced out of the lungs.

## G.   DIGESTIVE SYSTEM

The digestive system functions to reduce ingested food mechanically
and chemically to a state in which it can be used by the body. This
process occurs in the alimentary canal, which is composed of five
organs: the oral cavity, esophagus, stomach, and small and large intestines. In addition to the alimentary canal, there are adjunct organs,
including the salivary glands, liver, gallbladder, and pancreas, which
assist in **digestion.** ◀

Food enters the oral cavity, where it is acted on by teeth and
saliva. The teeth function to break up food. Incisors are used for biting, canines for tearing, and molars for crushing food. The food bolus is lubricated by **saliva,** primarily produced in the parotid, sub- ◀
mandibular, and sublingual glands.

Saliva is transported to the oral cavity through a system of ducts.
In addition to lubricating the food bolus, saliva contains the digestive
enzyme **ptyalin,** which begins the breakdown of starches in the ◀
mouth. The tongue pushes the food bolus downward into the
esophagus, which is a long tube that connects the oral cavity to the
stomach. Food moves quickly through the esophagus, assisted by
waves of muscular contractions in a process called peristalsis. In the
stomach, food is churned and acted on by a variety of gastric enzymes and hydrochloric acid. Some absorption into the bloodstream
takes place in the stomach, although most of the absorption is conducted mainly in the small intestine. Residual waste products not absorbed into the bloodstream enter the large intestine, or colon,
where water is absorbed, and the solid waste products are conducted outward from the body.

The liver is an adjunct organ of the digestive system and is involved in the formation of bile, which is important in the intestinal
phases of fat digestion. The liver also metabolizes carbohydrates,

| Digestive System Organs |
| --- |
| Oral cavity |
| Esophagus |
| Stomach |
| Small intestine |
| Large intestine |

fats, and proteins for storage or energy use. The importance of the ▶ liver as a **detoxification** organ cannot be overemphasized. It detoxifies harmful chemicals that enter the body. Many drugs used in dentistry (eg, local anesthetics) are broken down in the liver.

## H. EXCRETORY SYSTEM

The excretory system functions to remove waste products from the body, thereby supporting the maintenance of homeostasis. Included in the excretory system are the skin, lungs, intestines, and urinary tract.

The chemical reactions that take place within cells produce certain waste products, such as water, carbon dioxide, and urea, as well as heat, which must be eliminated from the body. This elimination process must occur regularly, or cell functioning will deteriorate, causing eventual death of the cell. The skin, which is the largest organ of the body, functions to eliminate water and various salts through perspiration. As water is eliminated, it evaporates, cooling the skin and lowering body temperature.

The lungs function to remove the carbon dioxide and water excreted during respiration. The intestines, both small and large, rid the body of solid and liquid waste products. Solid waste products include cellulose, roughage, and nondigestible material. Liquids excreted by the intestines are bile, calcium salts, and water.

The organs of the urinary system include the kidneys, ureters, bladder, and urethra. The two kidneys, located behind the abdominal cavity on each side of the spinal column, function in the balance of osmotic pressure of extracellular fluids. In addition, the kidneys control electrolyte balance and excretion of metabolic wastes, as well as regulating the pH level of body fluids.

## I. ENDOCRINE SYSTEM

▶ The endocrine system is responsible for secreting **hormones,** which regulate metabolic functions of the body. Hormones are chemicals that are specific in action, continuously secreted, and generally slow-acting. Organs of the endocrine system include the pituitary, thyroid, parathyroid, pineal, and adrenal glands, the pancreas, and the gonads. The pituitary, located in the cranial cavity, secretes several hormones.

The adrenal hormones are released through the influence of the pituitary hormone ACTH. The mineralocorticoids stimulate resorption of sodium in the kidneys, which in turn controls fluid balance in the body. The glucocorticoids predominantly act in the regulation of metabolism of carbohydrates, fats, and proteins. The adrenal gland also secretes epinephrine, which affects all structures of the body innervated by the sympathetic nervous system and thereby reinforces its action (cardiac acceleration, vasoconstriction, and rise in blood pressure).

The pancreas, located in the abdominal group of cells called the islets of Langerhans, secretes insulin. Insulin promotes the use of glucose in cells and thereby decreases blood glucose concentration. Insulin is essential for the maintenance of normal levels of blood glucose. A marked increase in the level of blood glucose is known as diabetes mellitus and is caused by an inadequate supply of insulin

---

## Excretory System Organs

Skin
Lungs
Intestines
Urinary tract

---

## Glands of the Endocrine System

Pituitary gland
Thyroid gland
Parathyroid gland
Pineal gland
Adrenal gland
Pancreas
Gonads

in the body. The pancreatic hormone glucagon increases the blood glucose level. Insulin and glucagon work together to maintain a normal blood glucose level.

A variety of hormones have numerous effects on the oral cavity. For instance, the development and eruption rate of teeth can be severely affected if there is an imbalance in the release of thyroid hormones. The abnormal release of epinephrine from the adrenals can have deleterious effects on the oral mucosa and pulp due to vasoconstriction. In addition, the female sex hormones estrogen and progesterone can exert harmful gingival effects, especially during pregnancy.

## J. REPRODUCTIVE SYSTEM

Humans reproduce sexually. Fertilization is the fusion of the nuclei of the female egg and the male sperm. Once a month, an ovum (egg) is emitted from a woman's ovary and enters one of the fallopian tubes. The egg then travels down toward the uterus. If the egg is not fertilized, it degenerates and is discharged from the body. If it is united with the sperm, it becomes a zygote.

An embryo in its later development is known as a fetus. Various physiologic developments occur along the course of a pregnancy. The face begins to develop between the third and twelfth weeks, teeth begin to develop around the sixth week, and the heart begins to form at about the fourth week.

The embryo is nourished through the placenta, a membrane through which oxygen, food, and waste products are exchanged. During the final trimester of pregnancy, the fetus increases greatly in size and weight, and brain cells form rapidly. The fetus also acquires antibodies from the mother, and immunity is transferred. Birth takes place approximately 266 days after conception.

During pregnancy, certain changes occur in the oral cavity of the mother as a result of hormonal fluctuation. The gingiva can become smooth, reddened, and swollen. Increased pocket depth can occur, causing teeth to become loose. Drugs taken by a pregnant woman can have an effect on the developing fetus. For example, tetracycline taken during the last trimester of pregnancy can cause discoloration of the teeth of the infant.

It is particularly important to ascertain whether a woman is pregnant before radiographs are taken. The fetus is most vulnerable during the first trimester. If radiographs are necessary, the pregnant woman should be draped with a lead-lined apron and exposed to the least amount of radiation possible.

## Summary

- The organs of the lymphatic system include lymph nodes, tonsils, thymus, and spleen. Lymph nodes filter the lymph fluid and produce lymphocytes and monocytes which destroy microorganisms in the body.
- Swelling of the lymph nodes is called lymphadenopathy.
- Respiration is the process by which the oxygen required by each cell for the production of energy is introduced into the blood stream and carbon dioxide, a waste product of cellular activity, is removed.

- The alimentary canal is composed of five organs; the oral cavity, esophagus, stomach, and small and large intestine.
- Saliva contains the digestive enzyme ptyalin which begins the breakdown of starches in the mouth.
- The liver detoxifies harmful chemicals that enter the body. Local anesthetics are broken down in the liver.
- The excretory system functions to remove waste products from the body, supporting the maintenance of homeostasis.
- Metabolic functions of the body are controlled by the endocrine system. The endocrine system secretes hormones.
- Insulin is essential for the maintenance of normal levels of blood glucose.
- An increase in the level of blood glucose is known as diabetes mellitus and is caused by an inadequate supply of insulin in the body.
- Development of the face of the embryo begins between the third and twelfth week of pregnancy. Teeth begin to develop at about the sixth week of gestation.

# III.   RELATED BIOMEDICAL SCIENCES

## Key Terms ◄

| | | |
|---|---|---|
| *ACQUIRED IMMUNITY* | *EPINEPHRINE* | *NITROUS OXIDE* |
| *AIDS* | *GENES* | *PERIODONTITIS* |
| *ANTIPYRETIC* | *GINGIVITIS* | *PRESCRIPTION* |
| *BENIGN* | *LEUKOPLAKIA* | *SQUAMOUS CELL CARCINOMA* |
| *BIOPSY* | *MALIGNANT* | *VIRUS* |

### Basic Cell Structures

Nucleus—controls cellular functions
Mitochondria—cell powerhouse
Lysosomes—stores all digestive enzymes
Endoplasmic reticulum—transports cellular material
Golgi apparatus—modifies secretory products of cell
Centrioles—cell division
Vacuoles—maintain cell fluid balance
Cell membrane—defines cell shape
Cytoplasm—suspends cell components in gel-like substance
Cilia—flagella enable cell movement

## A.   CYTOLOGY

Cytology is the study of cells. The cell is the basic unit of life, and its morphology (structure) is composed of the following basic components:

1. The nucleus is considered the brain of the cell, and controls all cellular functions.
2. Mitochondria are known as the powerhouses of the cell. They are responsible for energy production and respiration.
3. Lysosomes are vesicles that store many powerful digestive enzymes. They process bulk material that enters the cell and are enclosed within a membrane to prevent the release of these enzymes and to protect the cell from self-destruction.

4. The endoplasmic reticulum is a system of membranes within the cell that functions to transport various cellular material.
5. The Golgi apparatus consists of groups of small membranes that function in the storage and modification of secretory products.
6. Centrioles are paired cylindrical structures that lie adjacent to the nucleus and have a role in cell division.
7. Vacuoles are fluid-filled sacs that contain food products and waste material. They play a part in the fluid balance of the cell.
8. The cell membrane defines the shape of the cell and permits certain materials to enter and leave the cell.
9. Cytoplasm is a gel-like substance in which the cell components are suspended.
10. Cilia or flagella enable cell movement by shifting the cytoplasm within the cell.

Cells have three major functions: respiration, reproduction, and locomotion. The respiratory process is carried out by a series of complex chemical reactions that produce the energy necessary to support cellular function. Mitosis is the process of cell division, specifically, a division of the nucleus and cytoplasm. The result of mitosis is the production of a second cell that contains identical genetic materials (chromosomes) to the original cell.

Chromosomes are filamentous structures in the cell nucleus and contain genes. **Genes** are the basic units of heredity and are capable ◄ of self-replication.

Deoxyribonucleic acid (DNA) is the basic carrier of genetic information in the cells. It is included in every cell of the human body.

Genetics is the study of heredity and patterns of transmission of a given trait (eg, blue eyes or brown hair) from parent to offspring. Examples of genetic manifestations are sex determination, blood type, hemophilia, cleft palate, tooth hardness, saliva flow, and missing teeth. Significant developmental and growth disturbances in the oral cavity often have genetic implications. Disturbances in the development and growth of teeth, bones, and soft tissues are an important aspect in the study of dentistry.

| Major Cell Functions |
|---|
| Respiration |
| Reproduction |
| Locomotion |

## B.  HISTOLOGY

Histology is the microscopic study of the structure of tissues. Individual cells that form an organ or specialized tissue are related and perform specialized functions. The four basic types of tissues are epithelial, connective, muscle, and nervous tissue. Epithelial tissues act as a covering or lining of a body system, and connective tissue supports or binds body organs together. Muscle tissue and nervous tissue are composed of highly specialized cells and serve to coordinate the motor and sensory functions of the human body.

| Basic Types of Tissues |
|---|
| Epithelial |
| Connective |
| Muscle |
| Nervous |

## C.  MICROBIOLOGY

The oral cavity contains numerous types of microorganisms that can be transmitted easily during routine dental procedures. The importance of recognizing potential dangers from pathogenic microorganisms is the responsibility of all dental staff.

Microbiology is the study of biologic microorganisms which can only be seen with the aid of a microscope. These organisms are either single celled or multicelled. Some are beneficial and others are potential pathogens to humans. The three major classifications of microorganisms are viruses, fungi, and bacteria.

**Viruses** are the smallest infectious agents, and contain a strand molecule of nucleic acid encased in a protein shell. Viruses are parasites that replicate only in living cells. There are animal viruses, plant viruses, and bacterial viruses, which are also known as bacteriophages. Examples of pathologic conditions caused by viruses include herpes simplex, influenza, pneumonia, hepatitis, and HIV. Antibiotic drug therapy is ineffective for the treatment of viral infections.

Fungi include yeasts and molds. They are widely distributed microorganisms that grow as a mass of branching, interlacing filaments containing nuclei and organelles. A common intraoral disease caused by fungi is candidiasis or thrush. Antifungicide drugs, such as nystatin, effectively fight some fungal infections.

Bacteria are microorganisms that appear in three basic shapes: rod-shaped, spherical, and spiral. Rod-shaped bacteria are called bacilli, spherical bacteria are called cocci, and spiral bacteria are called spirilla. Bacteria have nuclei and are enclosed in cell walls. They have the ability to replicate themselves, and some are motile. Common pathologic conditions caused by bacteria are dental caries, periodontal disease, and rheumatic fever. Antibiotic drug therapy is generally used to fight systemic bacterial infections. The tubercle bacilli is a resistant organism that is responsible for tuberculosis.

Normal microbial constituents of the mouth include fungi, such as *Candida albicans,* and bacteria, such as *Streptococcus mutans* and *Staphylococcus.* These microorganisms are not harmful in normal amounts. It is only when they proliferate and disrupt homeostasis that pathologic conditions occur.

| Classification Microorganisms |
| --- |
| Viruses<br>Fungi<br>Bacteria |

## Summary

- Cells have three major functions: respiration, reproduction, and locomotion.
- Genes are the basic units of heredity and are capable of self-replication.
- The four basic types of tissues are epithelial, connective, muscle, and nervous tissue.
- Three major classifications of microorganisms are viruses, fungi, and bacteria.
- Pathologic conditions caused by viruses include herpes simplex, hepatitis, and HIV.
- Fungi cause an intraoral disease called candidiasis or thrush.
- Bacteria are microorganisms that are enclosed in cell walls. Pathologic conditions caused by bacteria include dental caries and periodontal disease.
- Tuberculosis is caused by a resistant bacteria tubercle bacilli.

## D. ORAL PATHOLOGY

Oral pathology is a recognized dental specialty concerned with the disease processes of the oral cavity. A wide range of pathologic conditions may affect the oral and maxillofacial structures. These oral manifestations may appear as a variety of surface lesions and can occur on hard or soft tissues of the oral cavity and surrounding extraoral structures of the head and neck. Oral diseases often occur due to developmental disturbances, such as cleft lip or palate abnormalities. Other oral pathologic conditions can be caused by infectious diseases, nutritional deficiencies, systemic body dysfunctions, and abnormal growths that are cancer-related. Oral diseases may appear as ulcerated lesions, cysts, vesicles, or tumors and are classified according to color, size, texture, and location.

The dental auxiliary's role includes collection and recording of clinical data, which may include a description of any abnormal findings in the head and neck region. A basic knowledge of pathology is necessary to differentiate between normal oral structures and abnormal findings in the oral cavity. Recognition of abnormal conditions in the oral cavity is vitally important for the auxiliary for protection from infectious diseases that may be transmitted during routine dental procedures. Strict adherence to proper barrier techniques, including gloves, masks, and eyewear, is indicated whenever direct patient contact is made in the oral cavity.

**1.   Biopsy.** Specific pathology tests are performed by the doctor to distinguish **benign** (nonmalignant) lesions from **malignant** (cancerous) lesions. These tests may include a **biopsy,** which requires a minor surgical procedure to remove a small specimen of the abnormal tissue for further diagnosis.

**2.   Exfoliative Cytology.** Exfoliative cytology is a nonsurgical procedure that is performed by scraping the surface of the lesion with a moistened wooden tongue blade and transferring the specimen to a prepared slide for further definitive study under the microscope (Fig. 1–2).

### Biopsy

Minor surgical procedure to remove a small specimen of abnormal tissue for diagnosis

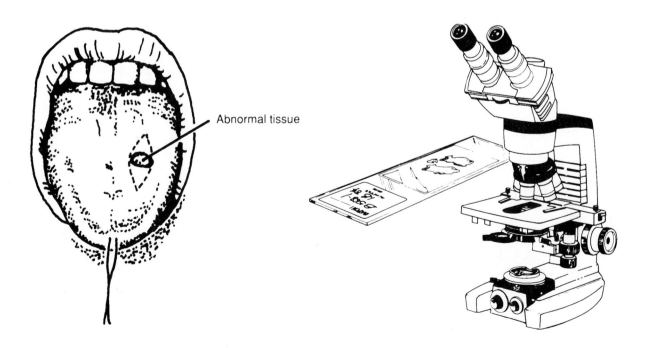

Abnormal tissue

Figure 1–2.  Tissue biopsy.

Both tests require the expertise of the oral pathologist for final diagnosis and appropriate treatment. All laboratory reports from the oral pathologist documenting the diagnosis of the oral lesion become part of the patient's permanent dental record.

## E. DISEASES OF THE PERIODONTIUM

**1.  Gingivitis and Periodontitis.** Periodontal disease, or pyorrhea, is one of the most widespread of all oral diseases. The most common periodontal disease is **gingivitis,** which is an inflammation of the gingiva, believed to be caused by products of microorganisms in plaque. Gingivitis is characterized by red, edematous, tender gingiva that may bleed easily. Gingivitis can be localized, involving only a small area, or generalized, involving the entire mouth. It can be acute or chronic. This disease is prevented by eliminating plaque through daily brushing and flossing.

When periodontal disease affects the alveolar bone, it is called **periodontitis.** It is usually painless and can result from untreated chronic gingivitis. Periodontitis may be characterized by inflamed gingival tissues that bleed easily, periodontal pocket formation, loss of alveolar bone, furcation involvement in multirooted teeth, gingival recession, and tooth mobility (Fig. 1–3). Advanced cases of periodontal disease may reveal abscess formation and exudate on gentle probing. Treatment of periodontal disease involves scaling and root planing and surgical procedures.

**2.  Acute Necrotizing Ulcerative Gingivitis.** Acute necrotizing ulcerative gingivitis (ANUG), also known as trench mouth or Vincent's infection, is characterized by ulcerations on the gingiva and a gray pseudomembrane. The diseased tissue may be localized or generalized. The characteristics of ANUG are pain, acute inflammation, bleeding, and sloughing of tissue between the teeth. In some patients, temperature is elevated and regional lymphadenopathy is present. The precise etiology of ANUG is unclear, but it appears to be related to physical and mental stress, smoking, and inadequate oral hygiene, which lowers overall resistance to bacterial infections. This

---

### Diseases of the Periodontium

Gingivitis
Periodontitis
ANUG—acute necrotizing ulcerative
    gingivitis
Pregnancy gingivitis

---

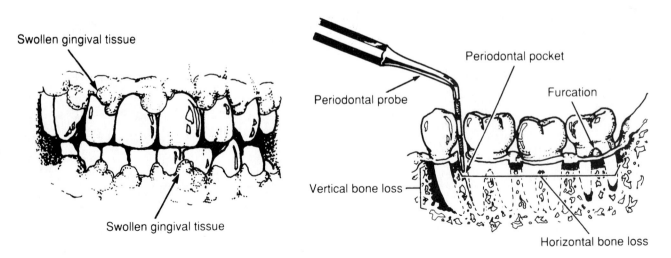

Swollen gingival tissue

Swollen gingival tissue

Periodontal pocket

Periodontal probe

Furcation

Vertical bone loss

Horizontal bone loss

Figure 1–3.  Gingival inflammation and periodontal involvement.

disease is treated by thoroughly scaling and rootplaning the affected gingival area and instructing the patient in proper oral hygiene home care.

**3. Pregnancy Gingivitis.** Pregnancy gingivitis is characterized by enlarged swollen gingival tissues that bleed easily. The condition is exaggerated by local irritants, such as plaque and calculus. The hormonal changes that take place within the body are also contributing factors to the gingival enlargement. Small benign growths, known as pregnancy tumors or pyogenic granulomas, can occur on the gingival tissues. The most frequent site of occurrence is the anterior incisor area of the oral cavity. Pregnancy gingivitis is treated by removing the local irritants through scaling and good oral hygiene. Most gingival tissues return to normal after delivery, but if there is no resolution, an excisional biopsy may be necessary.

## F.  DENTAL CARIES

Dental caries is a disease involving the hard structures of the teeth. Dental caries is responsible for the destruction and demineralization process that affects the enamel, dentin, and cementum. All age groups are susceptible hosts to dental decay.

There are several theories about the etiology of caries. A popular theory is called the acidogenic theory. It suggests that caries is the result of the activity of acid-producing bacteria. The process occurs as easily broken down carbohydrates adhere to teeth along with acid-producing bacteria in the form of plaque. The microorganisms cause the breakdown of the carbohydrates, resulting in the production of acids. When acidity in a given area exceeds a certain level, the inorganic tooth matrix is demineralized, and the organic matrix is destroyed.

A major cause of caries appears to be the refined foods present in daily diets. Refined softened foods tend to be cariogenic. Other contributing factors to host resistance include tooth shape, position, and composition, as well as the chemical composition of the saliva. Saliva is a complex fluid, the composition of which varies widely from person to person. Even within the same person, daily fluctuation is great. The pH level (ie, acidity) and the amount of saliva produced also are important factors. A decreasing pH level below 7, the amount of saliva, or both are associated with a tendency toward increased caries.

Treatment of caries is mechanical removal of the diseased tissue and appropriate restoration. If caries is left untreated, it will dissolve the hard enamel and subsequently affect the softer dentin of the tooth. Here, the caries spreads more quickly because the dentin has a higher organic content, which is easier to attack. Left unchecked, the process continues until the pulp is affected.

The dental pulp is a highly vascular structure, the primary function of which is the development of dentin during formation. Once matured, the pulp serves as a thermal sensor, a pain receptor and transmitter, and a supplier of nutrients. There are several causes of pulpal disease, including untreated decay, trauma, dental iatrogenic treatment, and exposure to chemical irritants. Pulpal diseases include pulpitis, pulpstones or denticles, and hyperemia. Pulpal infections also may include periapical abscesses.

**Dental Caries**

Disease involving the demineralization of enamel
Affects the dentin and cementum
Caused by acid-producing bacteria and refined carbohydrates

| **Developmental Pathologic Conditions** |
| --- |
| Anodontia—lack of teeth |
| Supernumerary teeth—excess number of teeth |
| Microdontia—small teeth |
| Macrodontia—large teeth |
| Gemination—division of tooth bud |
| Fusion—two teeth fuse |
| Dilaceration—sharp bend in roots |
| Amelogensis imperfecta—affects enamel |
| Dentinogensis imperfecta—affects dentin |
| Cleft lip/palate |

| **Lesions of the Tongue** |
| --- |
| Cleft tongue |
| Fissured tongue |
| Geographic tongue |
| Hairy tongue |
| Glossitis |

## G. DEVELOPMENTAL PATHOLOGIC CONDITIONS

In addition to those diseases that affect healthy tooth structure, there are a number of developmental anomalies. Anodontia, a lack of development of teeth, can be either partial or complete. A person can also develop an excess number of teeth, which are called supernumerary teeth. Teeth that are too small (microdontia) or too large (macrodontia) can develop. Additional disturbances that affect the shape of teeth include gemination, fusion, concrescence, and dilaceration. Gemination occurs during the attempted division of the tooth bud. Instead of the formation of one complete tooth, two incomplete teeth develop. Fusion occurs when two teeth partially or completely join or fuse, resulting in a single large tooth. If this process occurs after root formation and the cementum of two teeth is joined, it is termed concrescence. Dilaceration refers to the formation of roots with sharp bends or angles. Amelogenesis imperfecta refers to anomalies that occur during the formation of enamel, and correspondingly, dentinogenesis imperfecta refers to disturbances occurring during the formation of dentin.

The most common developmental pathologic state affecting the lips, palate, or both is a cleft, which appears as a result of lack of fusion. This condition occurs in approximately 1 in 800 births. If a cleft significantly interferes with the function of the oral or nasal cavity, surgical correction may be necessary.

## H. LESIONS OF THE TONGUE

The tongue also may be affected by developmental pathologic conditions, including cleft tongue, fissure tongue, geographic tongue, and hairy tongue. A cleft tongue results when fusion of the two halves of the tongue is incomplete. When an abnormal number of grooves or fissures appears on the dorsal side of the tongue, it is called fissured tongue. Benign migratory glossitis occurs when papillae on the tongue lose their surface epithelium. This is also known as geographic tongue because it may appear on different parts of the tongue at different times. A hairy tongue is characterized by an overgrowth (hypertrophy) of the filiform papillae. The tongue appears matted and may discolor, having a yellow, brown, or possibly black cast. Most of the developmental anomalies of the tongue are not clinically significant and are left untreated.

Nutritional disorders also may affect the tongue. Deficiency of vitamin B often results in a condition known as pellagra, where the tongue appears a bright scarlet red color, and is accompanied by a burning sensation. Glossitis is an inflammatory condition of the tongue with varied clinical changes in color and texture.

## I. COMMON ORAL PATHOLOGIC CONDITIONS

1. **Fordyce granules** are a developmental anomaly characterized by elevated sebaceous glands which appear in various sites in the oral cavity. They are small, multiple, yellowish spots, usually found on the buccal mucosa. Treatment is not necessary, since the granules are not pathologically significant.

2. **Tori** are bony protrusions appearing on the palate or mandible. They grow slowly and have no clinical significance unless they interfere with the placement of an oral prosthesis. If there is interference, tori are surgically removed. Torus palatinus most frequently occurs along the midline of the palate, and torus mandibularis occurs along the lingual aspect of the mandible in the cuspid and premolar regions.

3. **Abrasion** is the pathologic wearing away of tooth structure. This condition usually occurs in the cervical area of a single tooth or of several teeth. Abrasion occurs from excessive or improper toothbrushing or from the use of abrasive toothpastes. This condition is irreversible. Further damage can be prevented through patient education.

4. **Attrition** is the normal wearing away of the functional biting surfaces of the teeth by mastication. This normal process of tooth wear may be excessive because of particular personal habits, such as bruxism and the consumption of gritty foods. Bruxism is the unconscious grinding or clenching of teeth during sleep, often referred to as night grinding. Severe cases of bruxism can contribute to temporomandibular joint difficulties.

5. **Erosion** is the loss of tooth structure through a chemical process. This pathologic condition usually occurs on labial or buccal surfaces of teeth and can be related to the degree of acidity of saliva. Teeth may become hypersensitive. Clinical signs of erosion may be associated with nutritional and eating disorders, such as anorexia nervosa and bulimia. Stomach acids from repeated vomiting affect the enamel of the teeth, causing a decalcification effect similar to caries formation.

---

### Common Oral Pathologic Conditions

Fordyce granules—elevated sebaceous glands
Tori—bony growth on palate or floor of mouth
Abrasion—pathologic wear of tooth
Attrition—wear of biting surfaces
Erosion—loss of tooth by chemical process

---

## J. AUTOIMMUNE DISORDERS

Recurrent aphthous ulcers are commonly referred to as canker sores. In their early stages, aphthous ulcers are extremely painful and uncomfortable. Clinically, the lesions look like small ulcers and may occur anywhere in the oral cavity (eg, mucous membrane of lip, cheek, tongue, and floor of the mouth). They are sometimes associated with trauma or irritation, as from an ill-fitting appliance or denture. The exact etiology is unknown, although recurrent episodes of aphthous ulcers may be indicative of an altered autoimmune response of the oral epithelium or physical trauma.

## K. IMMUNITY

Infection is the process during which a microorganism enters into a relationship with the host, establishes itself, and multiplies within the host. The tissue environment controls susceptibility or resistance to given microorganisms. If the host lacks sufficient resistance, infection occurs.

Immunity is the property of a host to resist specific infections. **Acquired immunity** can be produced by an injection of antibodies ◀ of one person into another or by the formation of antibodies in a person as a result of previous exposure to a microorganism. Measles and poliovirus immunizations are examples of injected immunity. An acquired immunity to mumps or another disease results from a previous episode of the disease. The host may be born with natural antibodies against specific microorganisms, which is termed natural immunity.

## L. LESIONS ASSOCIATED WITH INFECTIOUS DISEASES

> ### Lesions Associated with Infectious Disease
>
> Herpes simplex—herpes, viral
> Varicella—chicken pox, viral
> Mumps—swelling of parotid gland
> Moniliasis—candidiasis or thrush, fungal
> Kaposi's sarcoma—AIDS
> Oral chancre—primary stage syphilis

1. **Herpes simplex,** commonly known as herpes or cold sores, is a contagious viral infection characterized by blister-like lesions that usually appear on the lips, but are found intraorally as well. Herpes is associated with severe sunburn, trauma, emotional stress, fever, and allergy. The disease is usually left untreated and runs its course in 7 to 14 days.

2. **Varicella,** commonly known as chickenpox, is a disease of viral origin in which fluid-filled lesions appear on the body. Occasionally, these small lesions occur intraorally.

3. **Mumps,** or parotitis, involves unilateral or bilateral swelling of the parotid and other salivary glands. Mumps is contagious and is usually found in children, although adults have been reported to contract the disease.

4. **Moniliasis,** also called candidiasis or thrush, is an infection caused by the fungus, *Candida albicans.* It is characterized by an elevated soft white plaque on the tongue or other oral tissues. Thrush appears in infants and debilitated persons. It has become more common in adults as a side effect of antibiotic medication, which tends to decrease other flora normally found in the oral cavity, allowing the fungal infection to dominate. Candidiasis frequently is associated with patients who have HIV infection. The lesions commonly occur on the palate, buccal mucosa, and dorsal surface of the tongue. The appearance is white to yellow and is curd-like in texture. When scraped off, the lesions leave a raw, bleeding area. Treatment may include application of an antifungal agent.

▶ 5. **Acquired immunodeficiency syndrome (AIDS)** is an infectious disease that attacks the human immune system. Patients who have been infected with the human immunodeficiency virus (HIV), which causes AIDS, are susceptible to various types of oral lesions and other opportunistic infections. Oral lesions frequently associated with AIDS include candidiasis, ANUG, hairy leukoplakia of the tongue, herpes simplex, and Kaposi's sarcoma.

6. **Syphilis** is a highly contagious disease, usually transmitted through sexual contact. However, the disease can be contracted through direct contact with the oral cavity of a person who is in an infectious stage. During the primary stage, chancres appear primarily on the genitalia, but can also arise on the soft tissues of the oral cavity. During the secondary stage, highly infectious oral lesions called mucous patches appear on the tongue, gingiva, or buccal mucosa. Tertiary syphilis is characterized by centrally necrotized oral lesions called gumma.

## M.  TUMORS OF THE ORAL CAVITY

Tumors are areas of swollen tissue often found in the oral cavity. It should be noted that the word tumor does not imply a cancerous or carcinogenic lesion.

### 1.  Benign Tumors

*a. Papillomas.* Papillomas are benign outward growths of surface epithelium commonly found on tongue, lips, buccal mucosa, gingiva, and palate. Papillomas are surgically removed only if they become uncomfortable to the patient or if they appear in areas that are easily traumatized.

*b. Pigmented Nevi.* Pigmented nevi, or moles, occur most commonly on the skin, but are also seen in the oral cavity. Moles are congenital anomalies characterized by brown pigmentation. Removal is recommended if they appear in easily irritated areas or if an observable change in color, size, or shape occurs.

*c. Fibroma.* A fibroma, or epulis, is an overgrowth of connective tissue that can result from infection or irritation. Fibromas grow slowly and are characterized by a change in color. They can occur anywhere in the oral cavity and are usually surgically removed.

*d. Hemangiomas.* Hemangiomas are tumors characterized by a proliferation of blood vessels. They vary widely in size and appear red or blue in color. Hemangiomas usually occur on the skin, lips, or buccal mucosa. They are clinically significant because they can hemorrhage if punctured.

*e. Pyogenic Granulomas.* Pyogenic granulomas are inflammatory overgrowths of unknown etiology. They are frequently seen on the gingiva and appear deep red or purple in color. They grow quickly and then remain static. Although painless, most are surgically removed. Tumors that are similar in composition often appear during the third month of pregnancy.

*f. Leukoplakia.* **Leukoplakia** appears as white patches or plaque ◀ occurring on mucosal surfaces. Unless infected, it is usually painless. The cause of leukoplakia is unclear, but factors related to its development appear to include tobacco, alcohol, irritations, vitamin deficiencies, and hormonal imbalances. Early diagnosis and histologic examination are important because leukoplakia precedes a malignant condition in 10% of cases. Treatment includes elimination of the irritating factors and surgical removal.

### 2.  Malignant Tumors

*a. Basal Cell Carcinoma.* Basal cell carcinoma occurs on exposed areas of the face and scalp, usually superior to the lower lip. It is characterized by small elevated areas that become ulcerated and is more prevalent in fair-skinned people. The most likely cause of basal cell carcinoma is overexposure to the sun. This tumor grows slowly and usually does not metastasize (spread). Treatment is surgical removal, with histologic examination of the removed tissue.

**Benign Tumors of the Oral Cavity**

Papilloma
Pigmented nevi
Fibroma
Hemangioma
Pyogenic granuloma
Leukoplakia

**Malignant Tumors**

Basal cell carcinoma
Squamous cell carcinoma
Melanoma

Prognosis for patients treated for this condition is usually good because of the lack of metastasis.

▶ *b. Epidermoid or Squamous Cell Carcinoma.* Epidermoid, or **squamous cell, carcinoma** is the most common form of cancer of the oral cavity. It can occur anywhere in the oral cavity and can have a different appearance in different areas. Possible causes of this disease include smoking, alcohol, nutritional deficiencies, syphilis, exposure to the sun, and viruses. Treatment for epidermoid or squamous cell carcinoma includes surgical removal, radiation therapy, and chemotherapy. These modalities may be administered either alone or in any combination.

*c. Melanomas.* Melanomas are often fatal neoplasms that usually occur on the skin and oral mucosa. Their appearance is similar to that of pigmented nevi, or moles, except that they have irregular borders and may have a history of rapid growth. Melanomas are uncommon and appear to be caused by trauma or irritation. Treatment is usually radical surgical removal followed by radiation, chemotherapy, or both.

## Summary

- A biopsy is performed by surgically removing a small specimen of abnormal tissue for further diagnosis. Exfoliative cytology is a non-surgical procedure.
- Gingivitis is a disease of the periodontium involving inflammation of the gums.
- Periodontal disease that affects the alveolar bone is called periodontitis.
- ANUG is also known as trench mouth and is characterized by ulcerated gingiva.
- A pregnancy tumor is called a pyogenic granuloma.
- Acid-producing bacteria in the form of plaque is responsible for the promotion of dental caries (decay).
- Pulpal diseases include pulpitis, pulpstones, hyperemia, and periapical abscesses.
- Most common developmental pathologic conditions include a cleft of either the lip or the palate.
- Recurrent apthous ulcers are called canker sores, and are a result of an autoimmune disorder.
- Immunity is the property of a host to resist specific infections.
- Lesions associated with infectious disease include candidiasis, mumps, varicella, herpes simplex, and Kaposi's sarcoma.
- Benign tumors of the oral cavity include papillomas, fibromas, pigmented nevi, pyogenic granuloma, hemangiomas, and leukoplakia.
- Malignant tumors of the oral cavity and head and neck region include squamous cell carcinoma, basal cell carcinoma, and melanoma.

## N. PHARMACOLOGY

Pharmacology is the scientific body of knowledge concerned with the properties of drugs and the interactions of chemical compounds within living systems. Drugs are classified as either proprietary (brand name), which are protected by a trademark, or generic (nonbrand), which reflects the products' chemical composition.

Drugs can be used as a means of sustaining and maintaining health. Examples of commonly used drugs in dentistry include antibiotics, sedatives, and analgesics. Antibiotics aid in the defense mechanisms of the body by inhibiting growth or destroying invading bacteria. Sedatives and hypnotics are examples of central nervous system depressants that can be useful in producing a calming effect for anxious dental patients. Pain-relieving drugs, such as nonnarcotic analgesics, assist in alleviating mild to moderate pain after dental procedures. Aspirin is an especially useful analgesic because it exhibits properties that are antipyretic (fever reducing) and anti-inflammatory.

The interaction of one drug with another might result in a deleterious effect on the patient. It is particularly important for an auxiliary who has taken a medical history to alert the doctor to any medication the patient is currently taking in order to prevent problems with medication interaction. For example, aspirin should not be prescribed for a patient taking an anticoagulant drug because these two drugs enhance each other's effect, and as a result, the patient could develop difficulties controlling bleeding.

**1.  Prescription Writing.** A **prescription** is a written order directing a pharmacist to dispense a certain drug with specific instructions to a patient. The dentist is the only member of the oral health care delivery team who is legally permitted to prescribe drugs.

A prescription contains the doctor's name, address, telephone number, and Drug Enforcement Agency (DEA) number. The patient's name, address, age, and the date of the prescription also are listed in the heading portion of the prescription order. The body of the prescription includes the superscription, or Rx symbol, which is an abbreviation literally meaning "take thou." The body of the prescription also contains the name of the drug to be dispensed, the strength, and the amount. Directions for the patient on how to take the drug are listed in the body of the prescription. At the bottom of the prescription order is information indicating whether a substitution for a generic brand drug is permissible. Refill information also is listed on the prescription form. The prescription must include the doctor's written signature. All prescriptions must be written in ink, and a duplicate copy or written documentation of the prescription must be recorded in the patient's dental chart for legal purposes. Figure 1–4 shows a sample prescription.

```
DEA #
            John Smith, D.D.S.
            Address
            Telephone

Name:                    Date:
Address:                 Age:

    RX
       Tetracycline USP, 250 mg
       Dispense: 30 capsules
       Signature: Take 2 stat and 1 q.i.d. subsequently


Refill _____      _____ D.D.S.
```

Figure 1–4. Sample prescription order.

Latin Terms and Abbreviations

| | |
|---|---|
| ac | before meals |
| bid | twice a day |
| c | with |
| disp | dispense |
| h | hour |
| pc | after meals |
| prn | as needed |
| qid | four times daily |
| tid | three times daily |
| stat | immediately |
| per os | by mouth |

## Methods of Drug Administration

| | |
|---|---|
| Topical | Intramuscular |
| Oral | Intradermal |
| Sublingual | Subcutaneous |
| Inhalation | Parenteral |
| Injection | Rectally |
| Intravenous | |

**2.  Methods of Administration.** Drugs are administered in a variety of ways, including topically (on the surface), orally, sublingually (under the tongue), rectally, by inhalation, and by injection. Injections can be given intravenously (into a vein), intramuscularly (into a muscle), intradermally (just breaking the skin surface), and subcutaneously (somewhat deeper than intradermally, into subcutaneous tissue). Parenteral administration refers to the introduction of medication in locations of the body other than the gastrointestinal tract.

Drugs are most commonly administered orally because of the relative ease of administration and low cost. A major disadvantage of drugs given orally, however, is that their potency can be diminished or eliminated by interaction with stomach enzymes, such as insulin. Sublingual administration produces rapid onset through the rich vascular network located beneath the tongue. Rectal administration of drugs is advantageous for patients with stomach disorders or for those who are unable to take a drug orally. Drugs administered by inhalation have a very quick onset. Parenteral administration has an almost immediate onset, but can be extremely dangerous if the drug is toxic to a patient.

**3.  Proper Handling of Drugs—Ordering and Inventory.** Careful records must be kept of all prescription drugs ordered for the dental office. This responsibility is often delegated to the dental auxiliary. Accurate inventory is required on a periodic basis to monitor and control the potential abuse of prescription drugs. All narcotic drugs ordered for the dental office must be ordered through the Bureau of Narcotics on special duplicate supply order forms. Narcotic drugs must be stored in a locked cabinet. When a narcotic drug is dispensed to a patient, the exact amount, date, and name of the patient must be recorded in the drug log book. Each entry must be initialed by the auxiliary. This information must also be documented in the patient's dental chart.

**4.  Storage of Prescription Drugs.** Drugs should be stored according to the manufacturer's directions. Certain drugs stored in the office emergency kit, such as nitroglycerin, must be monitored and replaced every 6 months, since they have a short shelf-life. Other drugs and medications must be kept out of direct sunlight and extreme temperature changes. Overexposure to air may cause a change in the consistency of the drug, consequently affecting the potency of the medication. Prevention of moisture contamination also must be considered. All caps or lids must be tightly applied, and well-fitted stoppers must be secured in bottled medications. Drugs that show changes in color or consistency or have reached their expiration dates must be discarded. All narcotic drugs that are discarded must be recorded on the drug log sheet. For security purposes, this procedure should be witnessed by two staff members and the doctor.

**5.  Telephone Procedures.** Prescription drugs are often requested by patients over the telephone. The dental assistant is not authorized by law to phone in a prescription for a patient. Inquiries related to prescriptions, such as dosage and refill questions, are often phoned into the dental office directly from the pharmacy. In these special cases, the dental assistant may provide this information to the pharmacist under direct verbal instruction from the dentist. Prescription refills conducted by phone must be followed up by careful and complete documentation in the patient's dental record.

## 6.  Categories of Medications

*a. Analgesics.* Analgesics (nonnarcotic) are administered to relieve mild to moderate pain. Mild analgesics include aspirin, acetaminophen (Tylenol), and propoxyphene hydrochloride (Darvon). Aspirin, in addition to being an analgesic, has **antipyretic** (fever-reducing) and anti-inflammatory properties. ◀

More potent analgesics are available only by prescription and include codeine, opiate, and synthetic opiate compounds. These drugs are sometimes prescribed for patients who have experienced painful procedures, such as extractions or complicated surgical procedures.

*b. Local Anesthesia.* Local anesthesia, administered by injection, causes a short-term reversible loss of sensation in a specific area of the body. Common local anesthetics include procaine (Novocain), lidocaine (Xylocaine), and mepivacaine (Carbocaine). Some local anesthetics contain vasoconstrictors, such as epinephrine, which prevent systemic absorption, thereby making the anesthetic longer-acting in the specific area. **Epinephrine,** which dilates bronchial ◀ muscles and increases the activity of the heart, is administered to patients who show evidence of severe allergic reaction or anaphylactic shock.

*c. Anesthetics.* Anesthetics are either general or local. General anesthetics induce sleep, eliminate noxious reflexes, and relax muscles. General anesthetics are administered intravenously or by inhalation methods. Intravenous drugs used for surgical procedures include methohexital sodium (Brevital) and thiopental sodium (Pentothal). Inhalation agents used for general anesthesia may include Halothane and Enflurane. A thorough explanation of preoperative instructions is required for dental patients undergoing general anesthesia. Postoperative responsibilities include close monitoring of vital signs and an adequate recovery period, with close supervision of the patient by the dental auxiliary.

*d. Nitrous Oxide.* Analgesia is the first stage of anesthesia, during which a patient remains conscious, has an increased threshold for

## Categories of Medications

| | |
|---|---|
| Analgesics | Antifungal |
| Anesthetics | Antihistamine |
| • General | CNS depressants |
| • Local | CNS stimulants |
| Nitrous oxide | Narcotics |
| Antibiotics | |

pain, and may experience some amnesia. Drugs commonly used for intravenous conscious sedation include diazepam (Valium) and meperidine hydrochloride (Demerol). **Nitrous oxide** and oxygen analgesia are administered by inhalation methods and are commonly used for various types of dental procedures.

Nitrous oxide may be used in conjunction with intravenous sedation and is beneficial for patients who are anxious or apprehensive. Hypertensive and cardiac patients may also benefit from nitrous oxide administration because it reduces stress and produces a higher concentration of oxygen.

Precautions and contraindications must be considered when administering any type of drug. Avoidance of prolonged nitrous oxide administration or high intake of the gas will reduce the potential for nausea and dizziness. Contraindications for nitrous oxide administration include nasal obstructions, pregnancy, and difficulty in communication of reflex and mood changes in a patient during the induction phase of nitrous oxide administration.

Nitrous oxide is effective primarily through the replacement of nitrogen in the bloodstream and must be administered with oxygen. Effective sedation may be reached with concentrations of nitrous oxide as low as 15% or as high as 50% depending on the patient and type of dental procedure performed. Nitrous oxide is a sweet-smelling gas that is nonflammable.

*e. Antibiotics.* Antibiotics are organic substances that destroy or inhibit the growth of bacteria. These drugs are used to prevent or alleviate bacterial infections. Penicillin is a bactericidal antibiotic that kills a wide range of microorganisms. Amoxicillin V is the most frequently prescribed antibiotic in dentistry for preventing bacteremias.

Some patients may have existing medical conditions that require antibiotics to be given prophylactically to prevent dangerous infections that could prove fatal. The patient's physician should be consulted before dental treatment in all questionable cases. Erythromycin and tetracycline are bacteriostatic antibiotics often prescribed for patients who are allergic to penicillin or Amoxicillin V.

*f. Antifungal Agents.* Antifungal agents are administered for treatment of fungal infections of the oral cavity. Nystatin is commonly used as an oral suspension to treat *Candida albicans* in cases of thrush.

*g. Antihistamines.* Antihistamines are effective in cases of severe allergic reactions. These drugs may produce several side effects, including drowsiness and xerostomia.

*h. Central Nervous System Depressants.* These include barbiturates, which are sedative hypnotics principally used to induce sleep, reduce anxiety, and alleviate convulsions. Common barbiturates are phenobarbital, secobarbital, and pentobarbital. Barbiturates should be dispensed with caution, however, since abuse can lead to respiratory depression, and result in coma or death. Patients should be told that mixing alcohol with barbiturates is particularly dangerous. Antianxiety drugs, such as diazepam (Valium) and chlordiazepoxide (Librium), are similar in action to barbiturates but are less potent.

*i. Central Nervous System Stimulants.* These include caffeine, epinephrine, and amphetamines. Caffeine contained in coffee, tea, and chocolate affects the cerebral cortex and causes restlessness and alertness. Epinephrine is contained in many local anesthetics because of its vasoconstrictive properties. Amphetamines are psychomotor stimulants and mood elevators, the disadvantages of which include a mild to moderate letdown after the initial stimulation. Central nervous system stimulants are rarely prescribed by dentists.

*j. Narcotics.* Narcotics are potent analgesics (pain-relieving drugs) derived from natural opiates or synthetic compounds. Common narcotics include codeine, meperidine (Demerol), and morphine. These drugs greatly elevate the pain threshold and are prescribed for moderate to severe pain. Toxic doses of narcotics can cause marked respiratory depression. Furthermore, if abused, dependency can occur. Other types of narcotic drugs may cause aggressiveness or rapid speech. The dental staff should observe each patient for possible signs and symptoms of drug abuse. Patients under the influence of drugs may exhibit irrational or unusual behavior patterns that must be handled appropriately to avoid injury to the patient or dental staff.

## Summary

- Drugs are classified as either proprietary (brand name) or generic (nonbrand).
- Aspirin is a useful analgesic which exhibits properties that are antipyretic (fever reducing) and anti-inflammatory.
- A prescription is a written order directing a pharmacist to dispense a certain drug with specific instructions to a patient.
- Drugs are more commonly administered orally.
- Inventory records must be kept of all prescription drugs ordered for the dental office.
- Drugs must be stored according to the manufacturer's directions.
- Nitroglycerin, if stored in the office emergency kit, must be replaced every six months.
- The dental auxiliary is not authorized by law to phone in a prescription for a patient.
- Local anesthetics contain vasoconstrictors such as epinephrine.
- General anesthetics induce sleep, eliminate noxious reflexes, and relax muscles.
- Nitrous oxide is beneficial for patients who are anxious or apprehensive.
- Antibiotics destroy or inhibit the growth of bacteria.
- Antihistamines are effective in cases of severe allergic reactions.
- Central nervous system depressants include barbiturates, which are sedative hypnotics.
- Central nervous system stimulants include epinephrine and caffeine.
- Narcotics are potent analgesics derived from natural opiates or synthetic compounds.

# Review Questions

1. Describe the basic structures of the cell.

2. What are the three major functions of a cell?

3. Name the four basic types of tissues in the human body.

4. What is the function of bone marrow?

5. List the three basic types of joints found in the skeletal system.

6. Distinguish between the three basic types of muscle in the muscular system.

7. Name the two major segments of the nervous system.

8. List the 12 paired cranial nerves and describe their function.

9. Describe functions of the components of the circulatory system. The following should be included in your description:

   • heart

   • blood vessels, arteries, veins, capillaries

   • blood

   • red blood cells

   • white blood cells

   • platelets

10. Explain how the lymphatic system plays an integral part in the body's defense systems.

11. Identify and locate the lymph nodes of the head and neck.

12. What is the primary function of the respiratory system?

13. Describe the digestive process and the functions of the organs of the alimentary canal. The following should be included in your description:

    • salivary glands

    • liver

    • gallbladder

    • pancreas

14. Discuss how hormones regulate the metabolic functions of the body.

15. How does the pancreas function within the endocrine system?

16. Describe the function of the excretory system.

17. Explain how the oral cavity soft and hard tissues may be affected during pregnancy.

18. Define the terms cytology and histology.

19. Name the three major classifications of microorganisms.

20. Identify the pathologic tests used by the doctor to distinguish between benign and malignant lesions.

21. Describe the characteristic clinical signs of the following:

    • gingivitis

- periodontitis

- ANUG

- pregnancy gingivitis

22. Discuss the acidogenic theory and the process of dental caries.

23. Identify the following developmental pathologic conditions:

- amelogensis imperfecta

- anodontia

- cleft lip/palate

- concrescence

- dentinogensis imperfecta

- dilaceration

- fusion

- gemination

- macrodontia

- microdontia

- supernumerary teeth

24. Describe the following common oral pathologic conditions:

- abrasion

- attrition

- erosion

- fordyce granules

- tori

25. Explain how immunity is acquired.

26. Identify six lesions associated with infectious diseases.

27. List six benign tumors and describe their clinical appearance.

28. What is the most common form of cancer of the oral cavity?

29. Name the two ways in which drugs are classified.

30. Identify the components of a prescription.

31. Describe the following methods of drug administration:

- oral

- topical

- sublingual

- inhalation

- intravenous

32. Discuss office protocol regarding prescription drug requests by patients over the telephone.

33. Give examples of the following drug categories and their effects on a patient:

- analgesics

- antibiotics

- antihistamines

- local anesthetics

- general anesthetics

- antifungal agents

- CNS stimulants

- CNS depressants

- narcotics

34. Explain indications and contraindications for the use of nitrous oxide.

# Dental Anatomy

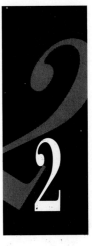

## Key Terms ◀

| | | |
|---|---|---|
| CALCIFICATION | INCISORS | PERIODONTIUM |
| CANINE | MANDIBLE | PREMOLAR |
| CRANIUM | MAXILLA | SUCCEDANEOUS |
| EXFOLIATE | MOLAR | TRIGEMINAL NERVE |
| GINGIVA | OCCLUSION | TEMPOROMANDIBULAR JOINT |

## I.  INTRODUCTION

A dental assistant must be aware of the fundamentals of head and neck anatomy, oral embryology, and tooth morphology in order to perform delegated dental procedures with a better understanding. This chapter presents the basic hard and soft tissue anatomic landmarks of the skull and oral cavity. A synopsis of the development of teeth and individual tooth morphology descriptions of the permanent dentition are presented.

## II.  ANATOMIC LANDMARKS OF THE SKULL

The skull is a bony structure composed of 22 bones. It is divided into the **cranium** (Table 2–1), which protects the brain, and the ◀

### Cranial Bones

Frontal (1)
Parietal (2)
Temporal (2)
Occipital (1)
Sphenoid (1)
Ethmoid (1)

TABLE 2–1. BONES OF THE CRANIUM

| BONES | ANATOMIC LANDMARKS |
|---|---|
| Frontal (1) | Superior anterior and roof of the skull; contains the frontal sinuses |
| Parietal (2) | Superior medial sides and roof of the skull |
| Temporal (2) | Medial sides of the skull; contains the middle ear, inner ear |
| Occipital (1) | Posterior base of the skull; posterior wall and posterior floor of cranial cavity |
| Sphenoid (1) | Anterior base of skull behind orbits |
| Ethmoid (1) | Part of nose, orbits, and floor of cranial cavity |

skeleton of the face. All the bones of the skull except the mandible are joined by immovable joints called sutures (Fig. 2–1).

▶ The upper jaw, or **maxilla,** contains the upper teeth. This irregularly shaped bone helps form the boundaries of the roof of the mouth, the floor and lateral walls of the nose, the floor of the orbit, and the maxillary sinus (Fig. 2–2; Table 2–2).

▶ The lower jaw, or **mandible,** contains the lower teeth. This horseshoe-shaped bone, the largest and strongest bone of the face, consists of the horizontal structure (body) and a pair of vertical structures (rami). Each ramus has two processes (extensions): the condylar process and the coronoid process. Soft tissue attachments (muscles and ligaments) to these processes enable the jaw to open and close (Figs. 2–3, 2–4).

▶ The range of motion of the mandible is defined by the **temporomandibular joint,** which is both a hinge joint and a gliding joint. This joint is a complex articulator composed of several ligaments that contribute to its functioning.

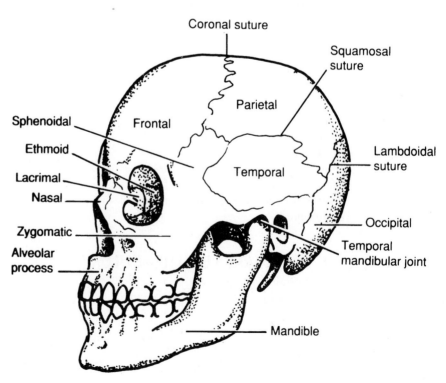

Figure 2–1. Bones of the cranium (lateral view).

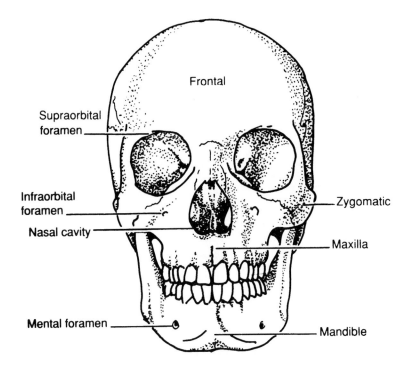

Frontal

Supraorbital foramen

Infraorbital foramen

Nasal cavity

Mental foramen

Zygomatic

Maxilla

Mandible

**Facial Bones**

Zygomatic (2)
Maxilla (2)
Nasal (2)
Lacrimal (2)
Palatine (2)
Vomer (1)
Inferior concha (2)
Mandible (1)

Figure 2–2. Bones of the face (frontal view).

TABLE 2–2. BONES OF THE FACE

| BONES | ANATOMIC LANDMARKS |
|---|---|
| Zygomatic (2) | Forms the prominence of the cheeks, lateral wall, and floor of the orbit |
| Maxilla (2) | Helps form the boundaries of the roof of the mouth, provides support for teeth of the upper arch; contains the maxillary sinus |
| Nasal (2) | Bridge of the nose |
| Lacrimal (2) | Anterior part of medial wall of the orbit |
| Palatine (2) | Floor of nasal cavity, floor of the orbit |
| Vomer (1) | Posterior and inferior portion of nasal septum |
| Inferior concha (2) | Lateral wall of nasal cavity |
| Mandible (1) | Consists of body, ramus, and angle; forms lower jaw and provides support for teeth; range of motion is defined by temporomandibular joint |

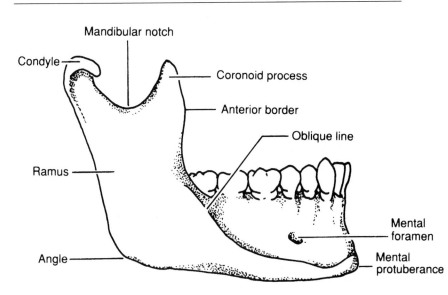

Mandibular notch

Condyle

Coronoid process

Anterior border

Oblique line

Ramus

Mental foramen

Angle

Mental protuberance

Figure 2–3. External aspect of mandible.

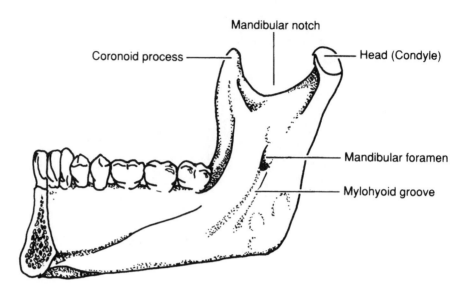

Figure 2–4. Internal aspect of mandible.

## III.   SOFT TISSUE LANDMARKS OF THE ORAL CAVITY

The oral cavity is the beginning of the digestive system. It is composed of the vestibule, bounded by the lips and cheeks externally and by the gums internally. The oral cavity proper is bounded by the alveolar arches, teeth, isthmus of fauces, hard and soft palate, and the tongue. It receives secretions from the salivary glands (Fig. 2–5).

The roof of the mouth is formed by the palate, which is divided into two areas: the hard palate and the soft palate. The hard palate separates the oral and nasal cavities and is bound by the alveolar arches and gingiva anteriorly and by the soft palate posteriorly. The soft palate is mostly muscular in origin and functions in speech and deglutition. Its posterior border hangs free and acts as a separation between the mouth and pharynx.

## IV.   THE SALIVARY GLANDS

The oral cavity contains three major paired glands that produce saliva. Saliva is a liquid medium that distributes basic digestive enzymes, lubricates the oral tissues and ingested food, and functions to maintain the balance of oral bacteria.

The parotid glands are located in front of and just below each ear. Their secretions enter the oral cavity through the parotid ducts (Stensen's), opening into the cheeks opposite the second maxillary molars.

The submandibular glands are located on the inner surface at the angle of the mandible. Their secretions enter the oral cavity through the submandibular (Wharton's) ducts located beneath the tongue in the anterior portion of the mouth (Fig. 2–6).

The sublingual glands are the smallest salivary glands and are located under the tongue. Their secretions enter the oral cavity by

### Salivary Glands and Ducts

Parotid gland—Stenson's duct
Submandibular gland—Wharton's duct
Sublingual gland—ducts of Rivinus

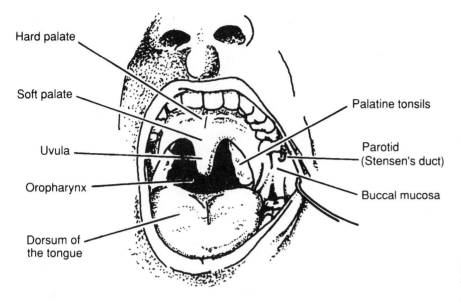

Figure 2–5. Soft tissue landmarks of the oral cavity.

the ducts of Rivinus. The secretions of the salivary glands are controlled by the autonomic nervous system.

## V.   THE TONGUE

The tongue functions in speech and mastication. It is also the major organ of taste.

The surface of the tongue contains several types of papillae, which contribute to its texture. Taste buds are located along the surface of the tongue and are found in large numbers in the papillae. Four basic taste senses are experienced: salty, sour, sweet, and bitter (Fig. 2–7).

## VI.   THE MAJOR MUSCLES

Muscles of mastication function in the movement of the mandible. Each side of the face has four major muscles: the temporal muscle, the internal (medial) pterygoid muscle, the external (lateral) pterygoid muscle, and the masseter (Fig. 2–8).

The temporal muscle closes and retracts the mandible. It originates in the temporal fossa and inserts onto the coronoid process and anterior border of the ramus of the mandible.

The internal (medial) pterygoid muscle closes the jaw. It originates on the pterygoid plate and inserts onto the inner (medial) surface of the angle of the mandible.

The external (lateral) pterygoid muscle opens the jaw and moves it both forward and laterally. It originates on the sphenoid bone and on the pterygoid plate and inserts onto the neck of the condyle and into the articular disc of the temporomandibular joint.

The masseter muscle closes the jaw. It originates from the zygomatic arch, and it inserts onto the lateral surface of the angle of the mandible.

The blood for these muscles is from the maxillary artery, a

**Muscles of Mastication**

Temporal
Internal (medial) pterygoid
External (lateral) pterygoid
Masseter

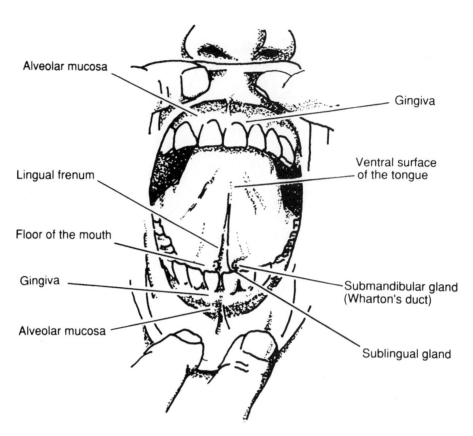

Alveolar mucosa

Gingiva

Lingual frenum

Ventral surface of the tongue

Floor of the mouth

Gingiva

Submandibular gland (Wharton's duct)

Alveolar mucosa

Sublingual gland

Figure 2–6. Oral cavity: salivary glands.

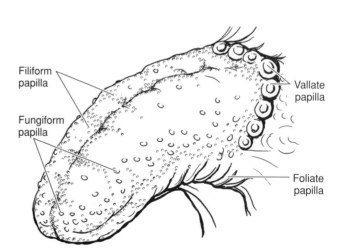

Filiform papilla

Fungiform papilla

Vallate papilla

Foliate papilla

Figure 2–7. The tongue (dorsal surface).

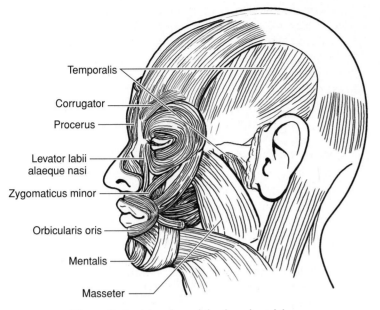

Figure 2–8. Muscles of the head and face.

branch of the external carotid artery. All the muscles of mastication are innervated by the **trigeminal nerve** (the fifth cranial nerve). ◀

Secondary muscles assist the masticatory process as well. These include the buccinator, the mylohyoid, the geniohyoid, and the anterior belly of the digastric muscle.

Muscles of facial expression are superficial muscles that have a tendency to relate to other nearby muscles and are grouped by the areas they affect. These basic groups affect the scalp, ears, nose, eyelids, and mouth. They enable expression and influence nonverbal communication. Blood is supplied by the external carotid artery, and innervation is supplied by the facial nerve.

## Summary

- The skull is composed of 22 bones. There are 8 bones in the cranium and 14 bones in the face.
- The upper jaw, or maxilla, contains the upper teeth. The lower jaw, or mandible, contains the lower teeth.
- The range of motion of the mandible is defined by the temporomandibular joint.
- The roof of the mouth is formed by the palate, which is divided into the hard palate and soft palate.
- Saliva is a liquid medium that distributes basic digestive enzymes, lubricates the oral tissues, and functions to maintain balance of the oral bacteria.
- Parotid salivary glands are located in front of and just below each ear. Their secretions enter the oral cavity through Stensen's duct.
- The submandibular salivary gland is located on the inner surface at the angle of the mandible. Their secretions enter the oral cavity through Wharton's duct.
- The tongue is the major organ of taste.
- Muscles of mastication function in the movement of the mandible.
- The temporal muscle closes and retracts the mandible.
- The internal (medial) pterygoid muscle closes the mandible.

## Muscles of Facial Expression

Mentalis
Orbicularis oris
Buccinator
Zygomaticus

- The external (lateral) pterygoid muscle opens the mandible and moves it forward and laterally.
- The masseter muscle closes the mandible.
- All the muscles of mastication are innervated by the trigeminal nerve (5th cranial nerve).
- Muscles of facial expression affect the scalp, ears, nose, eyelids, and mouth.

## VII.   ORAL EMBRYOLOGY

Teeth begin their development at approximately the sixth week in utero. The surface tissue of the oral cavity along the future dental arch thickens. This thickening tissue is called the dental lamina. Ten areas along the upper and lower arches possess further growth, causing the appearance of 10 swellings or buds, which are precursors of the future primary and later succedaneous (succeeding) teeth. The proliferating lamina leads to the formation of the shallow invagination of each bud into the oral tissue. From this, three distinct areas for each tooth develop. The first is the enamel organ, which is responsible for the formation of enamel. The second is the dental papillae, which is responsible for the development of dentin and pulp. The third is the dental sac, from which the cementum and periodontal ligament are developed. As growth continues, the teeth undergo a stage during which they all appear identical. This process continues until each tooth bud begins to differentiate into its final shape (eg, incisor, canine, molar). A period of apposition and **calcification** follows, during which enamel, dentin, and cementum fully mature. As each tooth matures, it begins to erupt in its appropriate place in the mouth.

Each person has two complete sets of teeth during a lifetime. The primary dentition begins to erupt around 6 months of age and is usually complete by the time a child is 2 years of age. This dentition is composed of 20 teeth: a central incisor, a lateral incisor, a canine, and a first and second molar in each quadrant. Primary teeth begin to **exfoliate** at approximately 6 years of age, when succedaneous teeth begin to erupt. **Succedaneous** teeth are the permanent teeth that replace primary teeth. This process continues until the child is approximately 11–12 years of age, when the exfoliation of the primary dentition is complete. Functions of primary teeth include the maintenance of space for permanent teeth, stimulation of growth of the jaws, mastication, and speech development. Primary teeth are different in size and in external and internal design from permanent teeth.

Succedaneous teeth continue to erupt until the child is approximately 12 years of age. With the exception of the third molars, the secondary dentition is complete. Third molars erupt between the ages of 17 and 21 years. Each quadrant in the permanent dentition is composed of a central and lateral incisor, a canine, two premolars, and three molars. In total, there are 32 teeth.

### Summary

- Teeth begin developing at approximately 6 weeks in utero.
- Tissue thickening of dental arches is called dental lamina.
- Formation of buds on dental lamina leads to development of primary and succedaneous teeth.

- The enamel organ forms tooth enamel.
- Dental papillae develops into the dentin and pulp of a tooth.
- The dental sac develops into tooth cementum and the periodontal ligament.
- Tooth buds mature and develop distinct shapes during the apposition and calcification stage.

## VIII.   TOOTH MORPHOLOGY

Teeth function primarily in the cutting and grinding of food. The shape of each tooth is determined by its function. Incisors are used for biting, canines for tearing, and molars for crushing food. Teeth also maintain the integrity of the dental arch, protect the supporting periodontal tissue, function in producing speech sounds, and are a component in each person's facial esthetics.

The teeth of the permanent dentition are divided into four general types: incisors, canines, premolars, and molars (Fig. 2–9). A description of each permanent tooth in the human dentition is presented for review.

**Types of Teeth**

Incisors
Canines
Premolars
Molars

### A.   *INCISORS*

**Incisors** act to shear or cut food and affect esthetics and speech. In the adult dentition, there are eight incisors, four in the maxilla and four in the mandible.

**1.   Maxillary Central Incisors.** The permanent central incisors erupt at 7 to 8 years of age and form the midline of the maxilla. The average central incisor is a single-rooted tooth that has a crown length of 10 mm, a root length of 12 mm, and a mesiodistal length of 9 mm at its widest point. This tooth is the widest anterior mesiodistal tooth. The labial surface is convex, but less convex than the maxillary lat-

Incisors          Cuspids          Premolars          Molars          Figure 2–9. Tooth morphology.

eral incisor. From a facial view, the crown of the tooth appears trapezoidal.

**2. Maxillary Lateral Incisors.** The maxillary lateral incisors erupt at approximately 8 to 9 years of age. The average lateral incisor is a single-rooted tooth that has a crown length of 8.8 mm, a root length of 13 mm, and a mesiodistal width of 6.4 mm at the incisal edge. The maxillary lateral incisor complements the function of the central incisor and resembles that tooth, except crown size and root bulk are smaller. Maxillary lateral incisors can exhibit more variation in tooth form than any other tooth except the third molar.

**3. Mandibular Central Incisors.** The mandibular central incisors erupt at approximately 6 to 7 years of age. The average crown length is 8.8 mm, root length is 11.8 mm, and the mesiodistal diameter is 5.4 mm at the incisal edge. These single-rooted teeth are usually the smallest permanent teeth and the most symmetrical teeth in the mouth.

**4. Mandibular Lateral Incisors.** The mandibular lateral incisors erupt at 7 to 8 years of age. The average crown length is 9.6 mm, root length is 12.7 mm, and the mesiodistal diameter is 5.9 mm at the incisal edge. These single-rooted teeth resemble the mandibular central incisors but are slightly larger in all dimensions.

## B. CANINES

▶ **Canines** are the longest teeth in the mouth. Like incisors, the function of these single-rooted teeth is to cut and tear food. There are four canines in the succedaneous dentition, one located in each quadrant between the lateral incisor and the first premolar. Since these teeth appear at the corners of the mouth when viewed facially, they have an important effect on appearance and esthetics.

**1. Maxillary Canines.** The maxillary canines erupt at 11 to 12 years of age. The average crown length is 9.5 mm, root length is 17.3 mm, and the mesiodistal width is 7.6 mm.

**2. Mandibular Canines.** The mandibular canines erupt at 9 to 10 years of age. The average crown length is 10.3 mm, and the root length is 15.3 mm. The mesiodistal width is 7.0 mm.

## C. PREMOLARS

▶ The adult mouth contains eight **premolars,** four in the upper jaw and four in the lower jaw. These teeth tear food and begin the grinding process and are located between the canines and molars. They succeed the deciduous molars.

**1. Maxillary First Premolars.** The maxillary first premolars erupt at 10 to 11 years of age. The average crown length is 8.2 mm, root length is 12.4 mm, and mesiodistal width is 6.9 mm at the incisal edge. The maxillary first premolars have well-defined buccal and lingual cusps. The buccal cusps are about 1.0 mm longer than the lingual cusps. The crowns are shorter than the canines but are similar in appearance to canines from the buccal aspect. The mesial surfaces of the teeth at the junction of the crown and root have a concavity. These are the only premolars with two roots.

**2.  Maxillary Second Premolars.** The maxillary second premolars erupt at 10 to 12 years of age. The average crown length is 7.5 mm, root length is 14.0 mm, and mesiodistal width is 6.8 mm at the incisal edge. The maxillary second premolars act in concert with the maxillary first premolars, and the two teeth resemble each other. The maxillary second premolars have one root as compared with the two roots of the maxillary first premolars, and the cusps of the second maxillary premolars are shorter than those of the first.

**3.  Mandibular First Premolars.** The mandibular first premolars erupt at approximately 10 to 12 years of age. The average crown length is 7.8 mm, root length is 14.0 mm, and the mesiodistal width is 6.9 mm. These teeth closely resemble the mandibular canines, since the buccal cusps are long and sharp, and the lingual cusps are not pronounced. They also resemble the anatomic shape of the mandibular second premolars.

**4.  Mandibular Second Premolars.** These teeth erupt at age 11 to 12 years. The average crown length is 7.9 mm, root length is 14.4 mm, and the mesiodistal length is 7.1 mm. These teeth appear with a buccal cusp and two smaller lingual cusps.

## D.  MOLARS

**Molars** perform the grinding job of mastication and reduce food to an appropriate size for swallowing. They are the largest teeth in the mouth in terms of bulk. There are 12 molars in the secondary dentition. Each quadrant contains three molars located posterior to the premolars.

**1.  Maxillary First Molars.** Average crown length of the maxillary first molars is 7.7 mm. These teeth have three roots; two buccal roots of approximately 12 mm length and a palatal root of about 13 mm length. These teeth are wider buccolingually than mesiodistal and are rhomboidal when viewed from the occlusal. There are usually four cusps, although there is sometimes a fifth cusp, located on the lingual surface, called the cusp of Carabelli. The occlusal surface is separated by a transverse ridge from the mesiolingual to the distobuccal cusps.

**2.  Maxillary Second and Third Molars.** The teeth supplement the action of the first molars. Second molars are very similar to first molars. The main difference is the lack of development of the distolingual cusps. Third molars often appear as a developmental anomaly, with considerable size variation. They are usually not as well developed as second molars, and, as a rule, the crowns are smaller and the roots may be fused.

**3.  Mandibular First Molars.** The average crown length of mandibular first molars is 7.7 mm. There are two roots, one mesial and one distal. Each is approximately 13.5 mm in length. In contrast to maxillary first molars, these are wider mesiodistally than buccolingually. Mandibular first molars usually have five cusps, three buccal and two lingual.

**4. Mandibular Second and Third Molars.** The mandibular second and third molars supplement the function of the first molars. Second molars are usually smaller than first molars and have only four cusps. Mandibular third molars vary considerably and are not usually as well developed as second molars. Their crowns generally follow the occlusal pattern of the other mandibular molars, but the roots are often small and not well-formed.

## Summary

- The shape of each tooth is determined by its specific function.
- Incisors are designed to cut food.
- There are 8 incisors in the permanent dentition.
- Canines have the longest roots and are designed for cutting or tearing food.
- There are 4 canines in the primary and permanent dentitions.
- Premolars are designed for tearing and grinding food.
- There are 8 premolars in the permanent dentition.
- Molars perform the grinding job of mastication.
- There are 12 molars in the permanent dentition and 8 molars in the primary dentition.

## IX.  OCCLUSION

▶ **Occlusion** is the study of how the masticatory system operates. This includes the placement of teeth in the arch, articulation, and the action of the supporting joints and muscles. The goal of oral health care is to maintain or restore the structural and functional harmony consistent with good health and comfort.

Common measurements used to describe occlusion include centric occlusion, centric relation, overjet, and overbite. Centric occlusion occurs at maximum intercuspation (tooth-to-tooth contact). Centric relation is a point determined when the mandible is in its most retruded position. This measurement is important when centric occlusion cannot be determined accurately as a result of missing tooth structure. Overjet is the horizontal distance and overbite is the vertical distance between upper and lower anterior teeth when teeth are in centric occlusion.

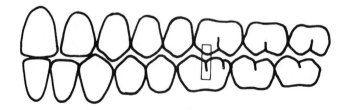

Figure 2–10. Class I neutrocclusion. Classification based on relationship of the first permanent premolars.

Determining proper occlusion is important in fabricating any dental restoration, since improper occlusion, or malocclusion, can lead to the unbalanced distribution of the forces of mastication and subsequently to more severe dental problems (Fig. 2–10).

## X.   THE PERIODONTIUM

The **periodontium** consists of those hard and soft tissues that support tooth function. It includes the gingiva, the alveolar bone, the periodontal ligament, and the cementum. The last three function to attach the tooth to the underlying maxilla or mandible.

The **gingiva** is the soft tissue that covers the cervical portions of the teeth and surrounding alveolar bone. It is composed of free gingiva and attached gingiva. The free gingiva extends from the gingival margin of the tooth to the bottom of the gingival sulcus and can be separated from the tooth. When measured with a periodontal probe, a healthy gingival sulcus will have a depth of 3 mm or less. The attached gingiva extends from the bottom of the gingival sulcus to the mucogingival junction.

At the base of the mucogingival junction, an alveolar lining mucosa that extends to the cheeks, floor of the mouth, and the lips continues. The alveolar lining mucosa is thin vascular mucosa and loosely attached.

The original margin appears as a wavy path from tooth to tooth, with the gingiva being highest in the interdental spaces. This tissue, which appears interproximally, is the interdental papilla (Fig. 2–11).

The tissue covering the free and attached gingiva is toughened through the process of keratinization and appears stippled. The covering of the alveolar tissue and sulcular tissue is not keratinized and can be damaged more easily.

Each tooth is connected to the underlying alveolar bone through an attachment apparatus. The attachment apparatus consists of the alveolar bone, the periodontal ligament, and the tooth cementum. It supports each tooth by suspending it in a sling mechanism. The periodontal ligament is the tissue enclosing each tooth and connecting the alveolar bone to the cementum. Cementum is a hard material similar to enamel and covers the root surfaces of each tooth. Alveolar bone is similar to bone found elsewhere in the body. However, the condition of this bone is dependent on the function of the tooth

**Periodontium Tissues**

Gingiva
Alveolar bone
Periodontal ligament
Cementum

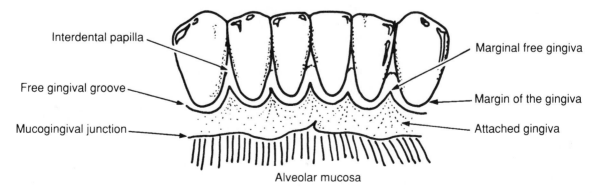

Figure 2–11. Periodontium: gingival tissues.

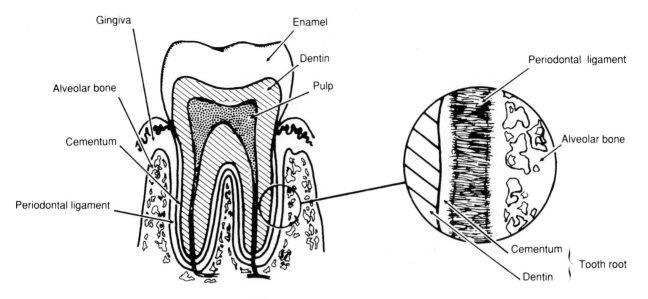

Figure 2–12. Periodontium: individual tooth and structures.

it surrounds. If the tooth is under high stress, the alveolar bone tends to become denser, whereas if the tooth is missing, the bone has a tendency to be resorbed by the body (Fig. 2–12).

A healthy periodontium is essential for the maintenance of oral health. It has become increasingly clear that most tooth loss during the middle and later years is caused by poor periodontal health and a general weakening of the periodontium.

## Summary

- Occlusion is the study of how the masticatory system operates.
- When teeth are in centric occlusion they are at maximum intercuspation.
- The horizontal distance between upper and lower anterior teeth is called overjet.
- The vertical distance between upper and lower anterior teeth is called overbite.
- The periodontium consists of those tissues that support tooth function, gingiva, alveolar bone, periodontal ligament, and cementum.
- A healthy gingival sulcus, when measured with a periodontal probe, will have a measurement depth of 3mm or less.
- The periodontal ligament encloses each tooth and serves to connect the alveolar bone to the cementum.
- Cementum is a hard tissue that covers the root surface of each tooth.
- The alveolar bone (process) provides a bony socket and support for each tooth in the maxillary and mandibular dentition.

# Review Questions

1. Identify the principal bony structures of the skull.

2. Explain the range of motion of the mandible.

3. Identify the soft tissue landmarks comprising the oral cavity and indicate their location.

4. Identify the three major salivary glands and their ducts.

5. Describe the three primary functions of the tongue.

6. Identify the four major muscle groups of the face.

7. Discuss the function of the superficial muscles of facial expression.

8. Discuss the functions of primary teeth.

9. Explain the process and stages of tooth development—oral embryology.

10. Identify the four general types of teeth of the permanent dentition and their function.

11. What is the relationship of the dental arches when in centric occlusion?

12. Name the hard and soft tissues of the periodontium.

# Preventive Dentistry

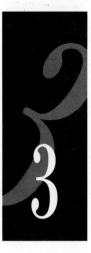

## Key Terms ◀

| | | |
|---|---|---|
| **BACTERIAL PLAQUE** | **FLUORIDE** | **NUTRIENTS** |
| **CALCULUS** | **INTERPROXIMAL BRUSH** | **PLAQUE CONTROL** |
| **DEMINERALIZE** | **INTRINSIC STAIN** | **RECALL** |
| **DISCLOSING AGENT** | **MATERIA ALBA** | **SEALANTS** |
| **EXTRINSIC STAIN** | **MOTTLED ENAMEL** | **SULCUS** |

## I. INTRODUCTION

Knowledge of disease prevention concepts and patient education skills is becoming mandatory for dental auxiliaries. The dental assistant must learn how to effectively motivate and train dental patients to assume greater responsibility for their own preventive treatment. Properly designed plaque control programs will assist patients in changing poor dental habits by providing new strategies for achieving dental health success. This chapter addresses the basic skills and concepts for preventing dental disease, including oral physiotherapy techniques, plaque etiology, nutritional counseling, **plaque** ◀ **control** programs, fluoride therapy, and the application of dental sealants.

## II.  SOFT DEPOSITS

### A.  BACTERIAL PLAQUE

▶ **Bacterial plaque** is a soft, sticky, dense, gelatinous layer of bacteria that adheres to the teeth and gingival tissues. Bacterial plaque is classified as a soft deposit and may be removed by proper toothbrushing methods and the use of dental floss, if accessible.

In the early stages of bacterial plaque formation, the pellicle layer is colorless and difficult to detect with the human eye. Later stages of plaque formation take on a thicker whitish appearance. Bacterial plaque is composed primarily of organized bacteria and salivary microorganisms held together in a sticky matrix.

The formation of bacterial plaque occurs rapidly in the oral cavity, and within 12 to 24 hours of removal, a thin film of bacterial plaque will begin to cover the teeth and gingival tissues again. Fermentable carbohydrates and sucrose in the diet increase the produc-
▶ tion of harmful bacterial plaque irritants (acids), which **demineralize** the tooth enamel, leading to dental caries. The irritants (acids) in dental plaque create gingival inflammation of the gums, causing gingival tissues to bleed and become swollen.

### B.  MATERIA ALBA

▶ **Materia alba** is a white or grayish mass of bacterial and oral cellular debris that accumulates around the gingival margins and on the surfaces of teeth. Materia alba is a loosely attached soft deposit that may be removed by vigorous rinsing or by water irrigating devices. The appearance of materia alba in the oral cavity is unesthetic and is associated with poor oral hygiene habits.

### C.  DENTAL STAINS

▶ **Extrinsic stains** are often caused by food, tobacco, coffee, or tea. The stains coat the outer surfaces of the teeth and can be removed by coronal polishing techniques. Extrinsic stains may range in color. Yellow and brown stains are often associated with food pigments and poor oral hygiene. Green stains may be caused by the remnants of Nasmyth's membrane around the newly erupted teeth of children. Orange and red stains are caused by certain types of chromogenic bacteria in the oral cavity as are black line stains, which occur around the cervical one-third of the tooth surface.

▶ **Intrinsic stains** can occur during tooth formation and are often caused by medication or systemic diseases. Intrinsic stains cannot be removed by coronal polishing techniques. The discoloration of the teeth may range from gray to black due to metallic materials coming in contact with the teeth. An intrinsic brown stain of the teeth, often
▶ referred to as dental fluorosis or **"mottled enamel,"** will occur if there is an excess of 2 parts per million of fluoride in the drinking water ingested during the mineralization stage of tooth formation. A common form of intrinsic stain is a result of ingestion of tetracycline during the calcification stage of tooth development. The discoloration may range from light yellow or gray to a characteristic darker gray banding around the cervical area of the teeth.

## III.  HARD DEPOSITS

If dental plaque is not removed, it may calcify. The result is a mineralized mass called **calculus.** Calculus is classified as a hard deposit and can be removed only by the use of dental instruments, such as scalers and curettes.

The accumulation of calculus above the gingival margin is known as supragingival calculus. This type of calculus is visible to the human eye. Supragingival calculus usually collects just above the gingival margin of the teeth near the ducts of the sublingual salivary glands of the anterior mandibular teeth and on the buccal surfaces of the maxillary second molars adjacent to Stenson's (parotid) salivary duct.

The formation of calculus below the gingival margin of teeth is known as subgingival calculus. Subgingival calculus is irritating to the gingival tissues and may lead to further gingival diseases due to plaque on and within the calculus matrix.

### Summary

- Bacterial plaque is a soft deposit that adheres to the teeth and gingival tissues.
- Bacterial plaque is composed of organized bacteria and salivary microorganisms held together in a sticky matrix.
- Plaque forms rapidly in the mouth and will reappear 12 to 24 hours after removal.
- Sucrose in the diet increases production of acids in bacterial plaque leading to demineralization of tooth enamel (decay).
- Plaque acids create gingival inflammation—gum disease.
- Materia alba is a loosely attached soft deposit associated with poor oral hygiene.
- Extrinsic stains range in color and may be caused by tobacco, food, coffee, and tea.
- The stains are removed by coronal polishing techniques.
- Intrinsic stains occur within the tooth and may develop during tooth formation. Intrinsic stains may also be caused by systemic disorders or medications.
- Dental fluorosis is an intrinsic stain also referred to as "mottled enamel."
- An excess of 2 parts per million fluoride in the drinking water may lead to dental fluorosis if ingested during the mineralization stage of tooth development.
- Calculus is a hard mineralized mass of bacterial plaque.
- Calculus is a hard deposit that can occur supragingival or subgingival.

## IV.  TOOTHBRUSHES AND BRUSHING TECHNIQUES

The proper toothbrush should be approximately ½-inch wide and contain two, three, or four rows of evenly spaced soft bristles. The tip of each bristle should be rounded, polished, and approximately 0.007 inches or less in diameter. The handle should be aligned on the same plane as the head of the toothbrush and provide a comfortable grasp to enable easy access to all areas of the mouth. Most

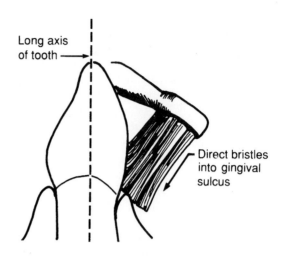

Figure 3–1. Toothbrush positioned for sulcular brushing.

common methods of brushing are the Bass, Charters, modified Stillman, and rolling stoke techniques.

## A.   BASS TECHNIQUE

The Bass technique emphasizes sulcular brushing and is the most effective method of brushing for removal of dental plaque deposits from beneath the gingival margin. The bristles of the toothbrush are placed at a 45-degree angle to the long axis of the tooth and gently placed into the **sulcus.** The brush is then vibrated back and forth with very short stokes for 10 to 15 seconds in each area (Fig. 3–1).

## B.   CHARTERS TECHNIQUE

The Charters technique was designed to stimulate the gingival margin around each tooth. It is most effective when interdental spaces are open. The bristles are pointed toward the occlusal or incisal surfaces at a 45-degree angle to the tooth. The bristles are pressed lightly in order to flex and force the bristle tips between the teeth. A firm but gentle vibrating motion is used. The bristle ends do not enter the sulcus.

## C.   MODIFIED STILLMAN TECHNIQUE

The modified Stillman technique is used to remove plaque from the cervical and interdental areas. The bristles of the brush are placed at a 45-degree angle to the apex of the tooth. The brush, lying firmly against the gingiva, is vibrated in a rotary motion. The wrist is turned slightly so that the brush slowly rolls down over the gingiva and teeth. A modified Stillman approach to brushing incorporates a rolling stroke after the vibratory stroke to ensure better plaque removal. With this technique, the bristles do not enter the sulcus.

## D.   ROLLING STROKE TECHNIQUE

The rolling stroke technique is the simplest. Bristles are placed at the gingival margin of the teeth with the side of the bristles pressing against the gingiva. The gingival tissues will be slightly blanched.

---

**Toothbrushing Methods**

Bass technique
Charters technique
Modified Stillman technique
Rolling stroke technique

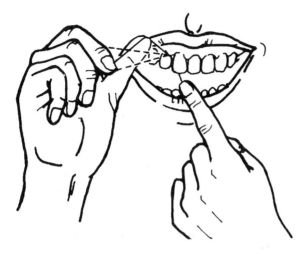

Figure 3–2. Flossing technique.

The brush is then rolled following the contours of the teeth onto the occlusal surfaces, and the process is repeated approximately 10 times on each tooth surface. Occlusal surfaces are cleaned with a back-and-forth motion. A disadvantage of this technique is that the sulcus is not cleaned.

## V.   DENTAL FLOSS AND FLOSSING TECHNIQUE

An important oral physiotherapy device for the removal of interproximal plaque is dental floss. Dental floss must be manipulated properly to avoid damaging tooth structure or gingiva. The interproximal areas of the teeth are the most frequent sites of dental caries and gingival inflammation, and toothbrushing alone is not effective in cleaning these areas. Flossing correctly may be difficult for the patient to learn. Each patient must be given sufficient support to ensure that the method is learned properly (Fig. 3–2).

A piece of floss, either waxed or unwaxed, approximately 18 inches long, should be wrapped around the middle finger of each hand until the fingers are about 2 inches apart. The floss is then guided interproximally with the thumb or index finger through the contact area with a short gentle seesawing motion. The dental floss must not be forced or snapped through the contact areas. Once through the contact area, the dental floss is pressed against the tooth and slightly curved to slide beneath the gingival margin until resistance is felt. While sliding the dental floss against the tooth surface, a scraping motion is used to remove the sticky plaque away from the gums and off the teeth. Various types of specialty dental floss are available for cleaning fixed bridgework and dental implants and require specific adaptation techniques for effective plaque removal.

## VI.   ORAL PHYSIOTHERAPY DEVICES

Several oral physiotherapy products are available to the dental patient for special dental health needs. Additional devices and products that can be used by the patient to clean the teeth and gums may include toothpaste, mouth rinses, disclosing agents, periodontal brushes, dental floss holders and threaders, wooden aids, and water irrigating devices. Specialty products for cleaning removable dental appliances and dentures also are available. These devices may include harder bristle toothbrushes, partial clasp brushes, denture toothpaste, and immersion agents used for cleansing and soaking removable partials and dentures.

## Oral Physiotherapy Devices

Disclosing agents
Interproximal brushes
Toothpaste—dentifrice
Cosmetic/therapeutic mouthrinses
Perio aids/piks
Rubber gingival tip stimulator
Floss holder
Wooden interdental wedge
Floss threader
Water irrigation devices
Partial clasp brush
Denture brush—immersion agent

## A.   TOOTHPASTE—DENTIFRICES

Toothpaste and dentifrices serve several functions. In addition to polishing teeth and decreasing mouth odors, they provide therapeutic benefits through the addition of fluorides to reduce the incidence of dental caries and desensitizing agents to reduce tooth sensitivity. Ingredients of toothpaste include water, which acts as a solvent; abrasives, which clean and polish; detergents, which provide foaming action; humectants, which prevent dehydration; binders, which join the solid and liquid ingredients; and flavorings.

## B.   MOUTHRINSES

Mouthrinses can be classified into two categories, cosmetic and therapeutic. Cosmetic rinses have no dental value that has been scientifically substantiated. Therapeutic rinses include the addition of fluoride for caries control and the addition of antibacterial plaque agents to promote healthier gingival tissues by reducing the oral microbacterial count.

## C.   DISCLOSING AGENTS

▶ **Disclosing agents** (tablets and solutions) are nontoxic, nonirritating, inexpensive dyes that identify plaque by coloring the deposits. Many deposits on teeth are not visible, and the tablets or solutions help the patient visualize these areas before or after brushing and flossing.

## D.   INTERPROXIMAL BRUSHES

▶ **Interproximal brushes** are cone-shaped nylon brushes used to remove plaque in open interproximal and bifurcated and trifurcated root areas. The brush is slightly moistened before insertion, and an in-and-out motion is used for cleansing. The plastic-coated interproximal brush is also an adjunct to hygiene maintenance of dental implants.

## E.   PERIO AIDS

Perio aids/piks are used to cleanse under the gingival margins and exposed furcation areas. Concave interdental surfaces also are best reached with the aid of the perio pik. The device consists of a plastic handle with a hole located at either end to insert the toothpick. The tip is angled and traced around the gingival margin to remove sulcular plaque deposits.

## F.  RUBBER-TIP STIMULATOR

A rubber tip is a cone-shaped piece of rubber used to stimulate the gingiva. The side of the tip is pressed against the gingiva with sufficient pressure to cause some blanching of the tissue and is then moved in circular motions. A rubber tip is useful in reshaping the gingiva after periodontal surgery, improving keratinization of tissue, and reducing the severity of interproximal inflammation.

## G.  WOODEN INTERDENTAL DEVICES

Wooden interdental devices are triangular-shaped wedges made of balsa wood. They are used for cleaning the interproximal areas where there are exposed tooth surfaces due to gingival recession. Care must be taken to use this device properly because gingival tissue may be traumatized if the adjoining teeth are forced apart.

## H.  FLOSS HOLDER

A floss holder is a device made for those patients who have difficulty grasping or manipulating the dental floss between their fingers. The floss holder is also a beneficial oral physiotherapy supplement for handicapped patients with limited dexterity. Care must be taken to avoid cutting the gingival tissues during application.

## I.  FLOSS THREADER

Floss threaders are plastic or metal devices used to thread floss under and between the pontics of fixed bridges and splinted teeth. These devices are important, since these areas are difficult to reach and are susceptible to plaque retention.

## J.  WATER IRRIGATOR

Water irrigation devices remove loose food debris around teeth. They are an adjunct, not a substitute, to toothbrushing because these instruments do not remove plaque. They are useful for patients with orthodontic and fixed prosthetic appliances. Proper attention must be given to the direction of the pulsing water jet to prevent injury to the delicate gingival tissues. The pressure of the water jet stream should never be set on high. Medications may be added to the water jet reservoir to enhance therapeutic results after mechanical debridement with the floss and toothbrush.

## VII.  FLUORIDES

The most efficient and economical method of decreasing the prevalence of dental caries is by the use of **fluorides.** Fluorides can be ◀ administered systemically, through addition to the water supply and vitamin supplements, or applied topically (directly onto the exposed surfaces of erupted teeth). Fluoride itself is a mineral nutrient essential in the formation of sound teeth and bones. However, if too much fluoride is absorbed during tooth developmental periods, the teeth can appear mottled.

## A. SYSTEMIC FLUORIDES

Many people receive fluoride in their drinking water in the amount of 1 part per million (ppm). If a community's central water supply is not fluoridated, individual community organizations, such as a school, can supplement their water supplies. In addition, fluoride supplements are available in the form of chewable tablets or liquids that can be added to a child's daily diet. Vitamins also may contain trace amounts of fluoride.

## B. TOPICAL FLUORIDES

Topical fluoride is applied directly to the surfaces of teeth and may be either an adjunct to fluoridated water or the sole source of fluoride for a child. Common topical fluoride agents include sodium fluoride, acidulated phosphate fluoride, and stannous fluoride.

**Sodium fluoride** is available in a 2% aqueous solution. A series of four treatments is given, with intervals of several days to 1 week apart.

**Acidulated phosphate fluoride** has proved more effective than sodium fluoride alone and is applied topically every 6 months.

**Stannous fluoride** is used in a 0.4% gel. Applications for root desensitization, caries control, or periodontal antimicrobial therapy may be prescribed.

Methods of application for topical fluoride gels may include disposable trays or trays that can be sterilized. Topical fluoride gels or solutions may be painted on the teeth with a cotton tip applicator. A summary of fluoride characteristics is outlined in Table 3–1.

Recommended amounts and methods of delivery for application of the fluoride agent must always be strictly followed. Dental auxiliaries should always keep patients in an upright position when administering a topical fluoride in a tray form. The patient should be instructed to keep a saliva ejector in the mouth to pick up excess flow of fluoride. Always caution the patient not to swallow immediately after the removal of the fluoride trays. The patient should be instructed to expectorate for several minutes after removal of the fluoride trays and then

TABLE 3–1. COMPARISON OF TOPICAL FLUORIDE CHARACTERISTICS

| FLUORIDE AGENT | ADVANTAGES | DISADVANTAGES |
| --- | --- | --- |
| Sodium fluoride (NaF) 2% | Does not stain teeth<br>Stable solution when stored in polyethylene bottle<br>Less objectionable taste<br>Gingival irritation does not occur | Success of treatment dependent on series of several appointments |
| Acidulated phosphate fluoride (APF) 1.23% NaF with 0.1 $M$ orthophosphoric acid | Does not stain teeth<br>Stable when stored in polyethylene bottle<br>Pleasant taste may be flavored<br>Requires single application | Can irritate inflamed ginvigal tissues<br>May cause etching effects on resin restoration or porcelain |
| Stannous fluoride ($SnF_2$) 0.4% | Available in liquid solution<br>May be incorporated in dentifrice for caries control<br>Brush-on gel form available for patient home use | Taste is objectionable<br>May cause staining of teeth<br>Short shelf-life<br>May be irritating to inflamed gingival tissues |

given proper home care instructions. Children should never be left unattended during the application of fluoride agents.

## C. FLUORIDE TOXICITY

Dental personnel must be aware of the potential dangers of fluoride toxicity. Failure to administer the correct dosage of prescribed fluoride agents may result in accidental overdose and serious injury. Signs and symptoms of an acute toxic reaction due to excess fluoride ingestion may include: abdominal pain, nausea, vomiting, and diarrhea. Cramping of the arms and legs, bronchospasms, and cardiac arrest may also occur.

Initial emergency treatment, if the patient is not vomiting, is to induce vomiting with a fluoride-binding liquid such as lime water or milk. Professional emergency support care should be sought as quickly as possible.

## VIII. DENTAL SEALANTS

Caries preventive treatment also includes the application of resin **sealants.** Pit and fissure sealants are caries-reducing agents that are applied directly to caries-free tooth surfaces to seal anatomic faults in the enamel of primary and permanent teeth. The most prevalent sites for caries are occlusal surfaces, where lesions usually begin in the deep pits and narrow fissures.

The tooth surface being treated is etched with phosphoric acid, and a resin sealant that mechanically bonds to enamel is applied and polymerized. This process results in the formation of a physical barrier which decreases the possibility of caries formation.

## IX. NUTRITION AND DIET ANALYSIS

Nutrition is the process that includes use of food in growth, repair, and maintenance of body tissues, digestion and absorption of food, and transport of food to the cells.

Good nutrition is a combination of basic food elements and chemical substances called **nutrients.** Nutrients are essential for providing the nourishment necessary for the body to function properly. Six general classes of nutrients can be identified: proteins, carbohydrates, fats, minerals, vitamins, and water.

## A. NUTRIENTS

**1. Proteins.** Proteins are made up of amino acids, and are either structural, serving as building blocks (eg, collagen fibers, the major constituents in skin, bone, and cartilage), or functional, including enzymes and hormones. Primary sources of protein include meat, poultry, fish, eggs, legumes, vegetables, nuts, cheese, and milk.

**2. Carbohydrates.** Carbohydrates (refined) provide sources of energy and include sugars (glucose, sucrose, lactose). Complex carbohydrates such as starches (rice, potatoes, grains), and polysaccharides (cellulose, roughage) provide energy, fiber, and additional nutrients. Carbohydrates are the principal energy source for most living systems and are the basic materials from which other molecules are built. Excess carbohydrates are stored in the liver.

**3.   Fat.** Fat serves a role both as a structural material and an energy reserve. It is important to the nervous system in providing insulation for nerves. Fats are found in meats, poultry, fish, oils, and dairy products.

**4.   Minerals.** Minerals are important in assisting enzymes in biochemical reactions. Essential minerals include calcium, sulfur, sodium, potassium, magnesium, iron, iodine, chlorine, and copper. Very small amounts of these minerals are needed to maintain adequate nutrition.

**5.   Vitamins.** Vitamins are organic compounds that are not synthesized by the body but are necessary for good health. Essential vitamins include A, B, C, D, E, and K.

**6.   Water.** Water is essential for all organisms and constitutes 50% to 70% of total body weight. Without water, we become dehydrated—a minor problem initially but one that can lead to serious complications and possibly death.

## B.   FOOD GROUPS

Good nutrition is essential for the maintenance of oral hygiene. Dietary counseling is given to patients to provide them with the knowledge necessary to maintain a dietary balance. Five food groups provide the sources for a balanced diet. The five food groups recommended for daily intake include the following.

**1.   Milk, Yogurt, & Cheese Group.** The milk group includes dairy products consisting of different types of milk, yogurt, cheese, ice cream, custards, and puddings that are an excellent source of protein, riboflavin, and calcium. The recommended daily allowance (RDA) for adults is 2–3 servings per day and for children three or more servings per day. For pregnant women, this amount is increased to four or more servings daily.

**2.   Meat, Poultry, Fish Group.** The meat group includes meat, poultry, fish, eggs, nuts, dried peas and beans, and lentils. Meats, poultry, and fish provide high-quality iron and B vitamins. The RDA is 2–3 servings daily.

**3.   Fruit Group.** The fruit group provides vitamins that are eliminated by the body and must be replenished daily. This food group also provides fiber and minerals essential to good health. Citrus fruits are a good food source for vitamin C, a water-soluble vitamin. Two to four servings a day are recommended from this food group.

**4.   Vegetable Group.** Three to five daily servings are recommended from the vegetable group. Vegetables may be cooked or raw. Dark green leafy vegetables are rich in vitamin A, a fat-soluble vitamin.

**5.   Bread, Cereal, Pasta, & Rice Group.** Breads and cereals provide vitamin B, protein, and iron. Sources include rice, pasta, whole

---

**USDA Recommended 5 Food Groups**

Bread, cereal, pasta, rice group
    Daily servings 6–11
Vegetable group
    Daily servings 3–5
Fruit Group
    Daily servings 2–4
Milk, yogurt, cheese group
    Daily servings 2–3
Meat, poultry, fish, eggs, nuts, dried
    beans
    Daily servings 2–3

TABLE 3–2. KEY NUTRIENTS

| NUTRIENT | FUNCTIONS | SOURCES | DEFICIENCY |
|---|---|---|---|
| Proteins | Build and maintain body tissues; help body carry on normal processes | Meat, poultry, fish, milk, cheese, eggs, plants (soybean) | Kwashiorkor, marasmus |
| Carbohydrates | Supply energy | Sugars, syrups, cereals, grains, bread, jam and jelly, pasta, crackers, pretzels, dried fruits | None specifically, but excessive intake can lead to dental caries |
| Fats | Provide insulation and support for internal body organs | Oils, butter, egg yolks, nuts, meats | None, but excessive fat intake can lead to coronary disease |
| Minerals | Assist in the formation and maintenance of body structures and metabolism | Milk, meat, fish, nuts, whole grains, shellfish | Bone deformities, muscle tremors, anemia |
| Water | Essential for maintaining normal body processes and stable body temperature | Drinking water and other liquids | Dehydration, shock, death |
| Vitamins | | | |
| Fat soluble | | | |
| A | Assists in proper maintenance of epithelial cells, plays role in vision | Fish, liver, oils, vegetables, yellow fruits | Night blindness, severe drying of skin |
| D | Builds and maintains bones and teeth, regulates calcium and phosphorus metabolism | Milk, fish, eggs, liver, butter, sunshine | Rickets, poor tooth development |
| E | Essential for normal reproduction | Wheat germ, vegetable oil, green vegetables | Unknown |
| K | Contributes to normal blood clotting | Green vegetables, cabbage, cauliflower, soybean oil | Defective clotting |
| Water soluble | | | |
| C | Aids in resisting infections, healing, and maintaining a healthy gingiva, strengthens blood vessels | Citrus, fruits, brocolli, parsley, green vegetables, melons, tomatoes, berries | Scurvy |
| $B_1$ (thiamine) | Helps normal body function growth, assists in carbohydrate metabolism | Yeast, wheat germ, whole grains, pork, liver | Growth retardation, nerve disorders, beriberi |
| $B_2$ | Contributes to normal function of body cells | Fish, eggs, whole grains, liver, meat, greens | Glossitis, cheilosis, dermatitis |
| $B_6$ | Contributes to normal function of body cells | Meat, liver, vegetables, whole grain cereals | Anemia, skin lesions |
| $B_{12}$ | Contributes to blood regeneration | Liver, milk, cheese | Pernicious anemia, neurologic disturbances |
| Niacin | Helps other cells use nutrients | Yeast, eggs, milk, green vegetables | Pellagra |
| Pantothenic acid | Assists in proper metabolism | Yeast, liver, kidney, eggs | Lack of proper metabolism |
| Folacin (folic acid) | Contributes to normal function of cells | Plant foods, greens, liver | Unknown |
| Biotin | Helps body use proteins, carbohydrates, and fats | Kidney, liver | Epithelial sensitivity, muscular pains |

grains, and enriched cereals. Nutrients are often lost during processing and are added later to compensate for this loss. Six or more servings a day are recommended from this group.

Suggested snack foods that aid in the maintenance of good oral health include fresh fruits and vegetables, cheese, eggs, nuts, lunch meats, fish, fowl, plain yogurt, milk, unsweetened juices, potato chips, popcorn, and sugar-free soft drinks.

Table 3–2 indicates the function and sources of key nutrients and disorders that can arise from nutritional deficiencies.

## X. PLAQUE-CONTROL PROGRAMS

Prevention and interception of dental disease occur only when patients have the knowledge and skills that enable them to participate in these processes. Educating and motivating patients to make a commitment to prevention is accomplished in a plaque-control program. Information is presented to patients to change their behavior in an effort to make them primarily responsible for maintaining good oral hygiene. A sample program follows.

### VISIT 1

Patients are made aware of how dental plaque forms. Basic instruction in brushing and flossing is provided, and disclosing agents are used to permit patients to see and remove soft deposits from their teeth. The relationship of dental plaque and dental disease is discussed.

### VISIT 2

Techniques of brushing and flossing are reviewed and reinforced. Adjunct oral physiotherapy techniques are introduced based on individual patient needs. Patients are provided with basic nutritional guidelines and a self-administered diet history review sheet. Emphasis should be placed on a low sugar and carbohydrate intake.

### VISIT 3

Diet history is reviewed, and constructive behavioral strategies helpful in changing poor eating habits are suggested. Home care is reviewed and evaluated. Corrections regarding technique are made at this time. Positive reinforcement is stressed to reward successes. Motivational strategies are emphasized and applied.

### VISIT 4

All previous sessions are reviewed for positive reinforcement. During this visit, patients are asked to describe or exhibit their individual strategies for prevention and to assess their own success. This visit may be repeated, if necessary, until success is achieved. The importance of future dental **recall** visits for preventive maintenance is reinforced. Long-term appointments may be set up at this visit also.

## Summary

- The Bass toothbrushing technique emphasizes sulcular brushing.
- Dental floss is used to remove interproximal plaque.
- Mouthrinses are classified into two categories, cosmetic and therapeutic.
- Disclosing agents identify plaque by coloring the deposit.
- Perio aids/piks are used to cleanse under the gingival margin and exposed furcation areas.
- A floss holder is beneficial for patients who have difficulty manipulating the dental floss.
- Water irrigation devices remove loose food debris around teeth.
- A floss threader is used to thread floss under and between the pontics of fixed bridges.
- Fluorides can be administered topically in a dental office or systemically through addition to the water supply.
- Fluoridation of the water supply is effective at 1 part per million.
- Failure to administer the correct dosage of prescribed fluoride agents may result in fluoride toxicity.
- Pit and fissure sealants are applied to the occlusal surfaces of caries-free teeth.
- Sealants are etched with phosphoric acid prior to application of the resin.
- Nutrition is a combination of basic food elements and nutrients.
- There are six key nutrient groups; proteins, carbohydrates, fats, minerals, vitamins, and water.
- The five food groups provide the sources for a balanced diet.
- Individualized plaque control programs assist to motivate the dental patient towards improved oral health.

# Review Questions

1. Explain how bacterial plaque is formed.

2. Describe how bacterial plaque causes demineralization of dental enamel.

3. What is materia alba?

4. List examples of extrinsic stains and intrinsic stains.

5. Discuss the formation of calculus, a hard deposit. How is calculus removed from the teeth?

6. Where does supragingival calculus primarily form in the mouth?

7. Discuss the importance of the sulcular toothbrushing technique.

8. Describe the method for using dental floss effectively in interproximal areas of the mouth.

9. Identify additional oral physiotherapy devices which are used for plaque control.

10. Discuss the differences between systemic and topical fluorides.

11. List signs and symptoms of fluoride toxicity.

12. Describe how a topical fluoride application is performed. Include pre- and post-patient instructions.

13. What are dental sealants? Discuss which teeth most often require sealants.

14. List the six key nutrients.

15. Describe the recommended USDA food groups and the daily recommended serving size.

16. Outline a four visit plaque control program including a recall visit.

# Infection Control

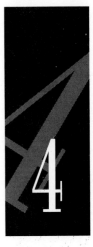

## Key Terms ◄

AEROSOL

ASEPSIS

BIOLOGICAL MONITORING

CROSS-CONTAMINATION

DECONTAMINATION

HIGH-LEVEL DISINFECTION

IMMUNIZATION

INTERMEDIATE-LEVEL DISINFECTION

PATHOGENS

PERSONAL PROTECTIVE EQUIPMENT

SEPSIS

SPORICIDAL

STERILIZATION

TUBERCULOCIDAL

UNIVERSAL PRECAUTIONS

## I.  INTRODUCTION

A primary responsibility of the dental auxiliary relates to the preparation and maintenance of an aseptic environment. Minimizing microbial disease transmission is a key objective in protecting the dental patient and dental health care worker. This chapter will present an overview of basic principle infection-control recommendations and guidelines. *To assist you in preparing for the Specialty Examination in Infection Control, it is recommended that you review Chapter 9, Occupational Safety–Bloodborne Pathogens Standard and Hazard Communication Standard.*

## II.  MODES OF DISEASE TRANSMISSION

▶ Infectious microorganisms may be transferred by various methods including direct contact, indirect contact, inhalation (**aerosol** droplets), contaminated food or water, and through cuts or breaks in the skin from an infectious vehicle source. The highest risk of infection transmission in the dental office is from the dental patient. Through direct contact with the dental patient during routine dental procedures, the dental team may be exposed to a variety of microorganisms from the patient's saliva, blood, and aerosol droplets inhaled at close proximity during treatment. Accidental needlesticks, sharp instrument injuries, or spatters of blood and saliva on the skin or in the eyes are examples of how a contaminated vehicle can be a source of infectious disease transmission.

▶ **Cross-contamination** can occur if appropriate methods of sterilization, disinfection, and waste disposal are not practiced. The spread of infectious microorganisms via the indirect contact mode of transmission occurs when dental staff touch other inanimate objects with soiled gloves or hands or by way of another contaminated vehicle.

Common examples of objects frequently touched in the dental operatory include dental unit light switch, operator's chair, operatory telephone, dental x-rays, dental charts, pens, and pencils. Each of these objects is a potential source of cross-contamination and serves to transmit infectious microorganisms to dental health care workers or to other patients.

## III.  UNIVERSAL PRECAUTIONS

▶ All patients must be considered potentially infectious when dental treatment is rendered. The term **universal precautions** implies that the same infection control procedures must be used for every patient. *Blood and saliva from all dental patients are considered potentially infectious materials.* The single most important measure to control transmission of hepatitis B virus (HBV) and HIV is to treat all human blood and other potentially infectious materials as if they were infectious for HBV and HIV. Application of this approach to infection control is referred to as Universal Precautions.

### Summary

- The dental health care worker may be exposed to a variety of microorganisms from the patient's saliva, blood, and aerosol droplets inhaled at close proximity during treatment.
- Cross-contamination can occur if appropriate methods of sterilization, disinfection, and waste disposal are not practiced.
- Infectious microorganisms may be transferred by direct contact, indirect contact, inhalation, contaminated food or water, and through cuts or breaks in the skin from an infectious vehicle source.
- "Universal Precautions" implies that the same infection control procedures must be used for every patient.
- Blood and saliva from all dental patients are considered potentially infectious materials.

## IV. MEDICAL HISTORY DATA

Patient medical and dental health history information must be reviewed prior to the beginning of each treatment session. The health status of each patient is determined by a health history.

Current questions relative to HIV and HBV should be included in medical/dental health history forms. Specific questions regarding recurrent illnesses with symptoms of unexplained weight loss, lymphadenopathy, and oral lesions may be asked either in interview or written questionnaire format. Medications and laboratory reports must also be noted. The patient's signature, date, and initials of the reviewing dentist should be documented in ink.

## V. HEPATITIS B VACCINATION

**Immunization** is the best protection against the hepatitis B virus. ◀ The HBV is found primarily in blood but can be found in other body fluids such as tears and saliva. HBV can also be transmitted through accidental needle sticks. All dental health care workers who come in contact with potentially infectious materials in an occupational setting should be immunized against the HBV.

## VI. PERSONAL PROTECTIVE EQUIPMENT & BARRIER TECHNIQUES

**Personal protective equipment** is specialized clothing or equip- ◀ ment worn by employees to protect themselves from exposure to blood or other potentially infectious materials. Personal protective equipment must not allow blood or other potentially infectious materials to pass through to clothing, skin, or mucous membranes.

In order to reduce the risk of infectious disease transmission in the dental environment, personal protective equipment must be used by all dental health care workers during patient treatment (Fig. 4–1).

Personal protective equipment includes the use of a disposable face mask, protective eyewear or face shield, and disposable gloves. Face masks should be changed at least once every hour and replaced more frequently if they become wet or soiled under heavy aerosol contamination. The face mask should cover the nose and mouth and protect against inhalation of pathogens during patient treatment. Placement of face mask is recommended before gloving.

Protective eyewear with sideguards should be wide enough to protect the eye, easily disinfected, and worn at all times during clinical procedures to protect eyes from flying debris and contamination.

Protective face shields should be used during clinical procedures that produce aerosol sprays. Use of the high-speed handpiece and ultrasonic scaling procedures produce aerosol sprays and release potential pathogenic microorganisms that can be inhaled. A face mask must be worn under the face shield.

Gloves must be worn by all staff members performing clinical patient care. The gloves serve as protective barriers for the dental health care worker and reduce the potential for cross-contamination in the dental office. Gloves that are torn or punctured should be dis-

| Personal Protective Equipment |
| --- |
| Disposable face mask |
| Disposable gloves |
| Face shield |
| Protective eyewear |
| Clinic jackets/lab coats |

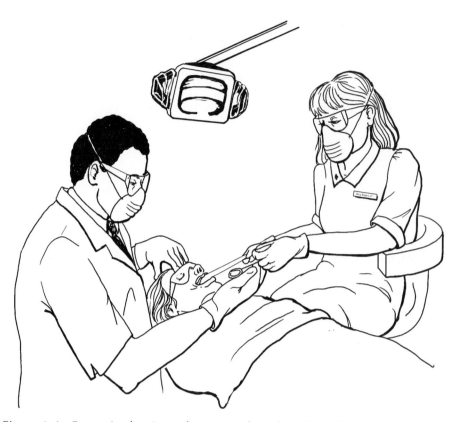

Figure 4–1. Protective barrier techniques reduce the risk of disease transmission.

carded and replaced with a new pair of gloves. Gloves worn for treatment or for examination must be changed between patients. Sterile surgical gloves are recommended for oral surgery and surgical periodontal procedures. *Always wash the hands thoroughly before and after removal of gloves.*

Gloves, clinic jackets, lab coats, and chin-length face shields, or the combination of masks with eye protection (such as glasses with solid side shields or goggles) must be worn whenever splashes, spray, spatter, or droplets of blood or other infectious materials may be generated.

Contaminated personal protective equipment must be placed in an appropriately designated area or container for storing, washing, decontaminating, or discarding.

Plastic or foil covers, used to protect surfaces and equipment such as light handles or x-ray unit heads must be replaced when contaminated. Surfaces not covered by protective barriers must be cleaned and surface disinfected with an approved EPA intermediate-level disinfectant.

Additional protective barrier techniques include the use of a rubber dam and high-velocity oral evacuation system to minimize the formation of aerosols during patient treatment.

## VII. HANDWASHING

Protective barriers for the hands include gloves and proper handwashing techniques. Before placing gloves, hands should be washed thoroughly with a liquid antimicrobial soap. All jewelry should be removed, since microorganisms may harbor under rings and watches. A soft sterile nail brush or disposable type sponge should be used to clean under fingernails. Nail brushes are cleaned and sterilized after use.

Surgical procedures require the use of a standard surgical scrub that is performed in a sequential order. Initial surgical hand scrubs take anywhere from 5 to 10 minutes. Hands, wrists, and arms up to the elbow are scrubbed with overlapping circular strokes and sufficient soap lather.

## Summary

- Patient medical and dental health history information is to be reviewed prior to the beginning of each treatment session.
- Immunization is the best protection against the hepatitis B virus.
- To reduce the risk of infectious disease transmission in the dental environment, personal protective equipment must be used.
- Disposable face masks should be changed for each patient and replaced if they become wet or soiled.
- Protective eyewear should be worn at all times during clinical procedures to protect the eyes from flying debris and contamination.
- Disposable gloves reduce the potential of cross-contamination in the dental office.
- Gloves that are torn or punctured should be discarded and replaced with a new pair of gloves.
- Gloves worn for treatment or for examination must be changed between patients.
- Sterile surgical gloves are recommended for periodontal and oral surgical procedures.
- Protective face shields should be used during clinical procedures that produce aerosol sprays.
- Protective barriers are used to cover surfaces and equipment such as light handles or x-ray unit heads.
- The high-velocity oral evacuation system minimizes the formation of aerosols during patient treatment.
- Hands should be washed thoroughly with a liquid antimicrobial soap.
- All jewelry should be removed, since microorganisms may harbor under rings and watches.

## VIII.  STERILIZATION

**Asepsis** is the term used to describe freedom from pathologic microorganisms **(pathogens).** Conversely, **sepsis** refers to the existence of disease-producing organisms. **Sterilization** destroys all forms of microscopic life, including bacterial spores and viruses, by chemical or physical agents. *All instruments that will penetrate soft tissue or come in contact with bone must be sterilized.*

Recognized methods of sterilization include dry heat, steam autoclave (moist heat), chemical vapor under pressure, immersion in a high-level disinfectant, and ethylene oxide. To determine which method of sterilization is appropriate for contaminated instruments, the Centers for Disease Control and Prevention recommends identi-

| Methods of Sterilization |
| --- |
| Dry heat<br>Steam autoclave<br>Chemical vapor<br>Ethylene oxide<br>High-level disinfectant |

fying items according to the way in which an instrument contacts patients (Spaulding modified classification system).

- Critical—Instruments that penetrate soft tissue or bone. Examples include dental handpiece, burs, scalers, and surgical instruments. Items require an approved method of sterilization.
- Semicritical—Instruments that touch oral tissues but do not contact bone or penetrate soft tissues. Examples include amalgam, condensers, mouth mirrors. Sterilization is required.
- Noncritical—Instruments that will not be used in the mouth but will come in contact with intact skin. Examples include the x-ray machine tube head. Items require low-level disinfection.

Dry heat ovens use heat alone to sterilize instruments and material. Sterilization cycles may last from 1 to 2 hours. The dry heat method of sterilization is effective for instruments that tend to rust or dull easily under other approved methods of sterilization.

Steam autoclaves (moist heat) use high temperatures to achieve sufficient pressure to generate steam. The steam under pressure method of autoclaving is preferred by most dental offices because of the shorter sterilization time cycles and the autoclave's effectiveness in destroying infectious microorganisms, including spores and viruses.

Chemical vapor sterilizers use such agents as formaldehyde, alcohol mixtures, water and acetone, or other related chemicals. Under heat, the sterilizer creates sufficient pressure to generate a gas that is an effective, recognized method of sterilization. The use of chemical vapor sterilizers requires adequate ventilation because of the release of potentially harmful vapors.

*Immersion methods of chemical sterilization are used when other approved methods of heat sterilization cannot be applied.* Dental instruments or materials that have been contaminated by the penetration of soft tissues or bone must be immersed for long exposure time cycles of up to 10 hours. Only products approved and registered by the Environmental Protection Agency (EPA) can be effectively used. High-level disinfectants must display a chemical label stating this "sterilant/disinfectant" EPA information.

After the sterilization process is complete, rinse item in sterile water, dry, and store in sterile container. Whenever possible, disposable (one time use only) items should be used. Sterilization monitoring methods that require spore tests *cannot* be processed using the immersion method of chemical sterilization.

Ethylene oxide sterilization methods involve the use of special gas sterilizers. Hospitals and institutions commonly use this form of sterilization. Ethylene oxide is an effective method of sterilization for most dental materials such as plastic, cloth, and nitrous oxide armamentarium, including rubber hoses and nondisposable rubber masks. The sterilization time cycle is long, averaging a minimum of 12 hours, with an adequate aeration time period following removal from the sterilizer. Appropriate ventilation is required when working with the ethylene oxide gas sterilizer.

## Instrument Classification (Spaulding)

Critical—instruments that penetrate soft tissue or bone.

Semicritical—instruments that touch oral tissues but do not contact bone or penetrate soft tissues.

Noncritical—instruments that will not be used in the mouth but will come in contact with intact skin.

## Summary

- Asepsis is a term used to describe freedom from pathologic microorganisms.
- Sterilization destroys all forms of microscopic life, including bacterial spores and viruses, by chemical or physical agents.

- Instruments that penetrate soft tissue or come in contact with bone must be sterilized.
- Recognized methods of sterilization include dry heat, steam auto-clave, chemical vapor under pressure, ethylene oxide, and im-mersion in a high-level disinfectant.
- To determine the appropriate method of sterilization for contami-nated instruments, classify as follows:

    "critical"—Instruments which penetrate soft tissue or bone.

    "semicritical"—Instruments that touch oral tissues but do not contact bone or penetrate soft tissues.

    "noncritical"—Instruments that will not be used in the mouth but will come in contact with intact skin.

- The dry heat method of sterilization is effective for instruments that tend to rust or dull easily.
- Steam autoclaves use high temperatures to achieve sufficient pressure to generate steam.
- Chemical vapor sterilizers use agents such as formaldehyde, alco-hol mixtures, and other related chemicals.
- The use of chemical vapor sterilizers requires adequate ventila-tion because of the release of potentially harmful vapors.
- Immersion methods of chemical sterilization are used only when other approved methods of sterilization cannot be applied.
- High-level disinfectants must be EPA approved and registered as a "sterilant/disinfectant."
- Exposure cycles for immersion methods of chemical sterilization may be as long as 10 hours.
- Ethylene oxide sterilization methods are used for plastic, cloth, and nitrous oxide rubber hoses and nondisposable rubber masks.
- The ethylene oxide sterilization cycle averages a minimum of 12 hours.

## IX.  STERILIZATION MONITORING

The CDC recommends weekly monitoring of dental sterilizers. *The three forms of sterilization monitoring include biological, chemical, or physical monitoring.* Monitoring is performed to assure sterility. **Biological monitoring** (spore-testing) provides the best means of verification for assurance of sterilization.

> **Sterilization Monitoring Methods**
>
> Biological monitoring (spore-testing)
> Chemical monitoring
> Physical monitoring

Biological monitoring may be done in-office or through a ster-ilization monitoring service which requires mail-in monitoring for the results of the sterilization cycle tested. Biological indicators are placed inside the chamber during processing in the center of the load. The biological indicator contains bacterial endospores used for spore testing. Biological indicators may be housed in self-contained spore vials, or paper spore strips in protective glassine en-velopes.

At the end of the processing cycle, the biological indicator is re-moved and incubated to determine if the bacterial spores were killed. A control biological indicator which is **not run through the sterilization cycle** is also incubated and analyzed along with the test biological indicator to confirm that if live spores are present they can yield growth.

## Biological Monitoring (Spore Testing)

Positive test results indicate sterilization failure

Negative test results indicate sterilization

If a **positive** biological indicator test occurs this indicates sterilization failure and the instruments processed should not be used. Corrective measures must be taken immediately to resolve the problem. A **negative** biological indicator test indicates sterilization.

Chemical monitoring uses heat sensitive chemicals in the form of indicators on autoclave tape, paper strips, labels, and markings on sterilization pouches or bags. There are two types of chemical indicators: the rapid-change indicator and the slow-change, or integrated, indicator.

The rapid-change indicator is used on the outside of a pack or cassette to identify that the instruments have been heat-processed. The rapid-change indicator *does not* assure sterilization. This method of monitoring demonstrates only that the instrument pack or cassette has been exposed to a certain temperature for the appropriate length of time to cause a color change in the chemical indicator.

The slow-change, or integrated, indicator is used on the inside of a pack, pouch, or cassette. The integrated indicator changes color slowly and responds to a combination of time, temperature, and steam.

*If there is no color change with either the external rapid change or internal slow change indicators do not use the processed instruments until corrective measures are taken to resolve the problem.* Spore testing should be conducted to assist in determining if the sterilizer is functioning properly.

Physical monitoring is performed by observing the gauges or dials on the sterilizers and recording the sterilizing temperature, pressure, and exposure time. Physical monitoring does not assure sterilization inside an individual pack or pouch of instruments. A combination of all three sterilization monitoring procedures should be incorporated into the daily dental practice for appropriate instrument sterilization monitoring.

## Summary

- Weekly monitoring of dental sterilizers is recommended by the CDC.
- The three forms of sterilization monitoring include biological, chemical, and physical monitoring.
- Monitoring is performed to assure sterility.
- Biological monitoring (spore testing) provides the best means of verification for assurance of sterilization.
- Biological monitoring may be done in office or through a sterilization monitoring service.
- The biological indicator contains bacterial endospores used for spore testing:

  A POSITIVE biological indicator test indicates sterilization failure.

  A NEGATIVE biological indicator test indicates sterilization.

- Rapid change indicators are used on the outside of an instrument pack.
- Slow change indicators are used on the inside of an instrument pack.
- If there is no color change with either the external rapid change or internal slow change indicators, do not use the processed instruments.

■ Physical monitoring is performed by observing the gauges or dials on the sterilizers and recording the sterilizing temperature, pressure, and exposure time.

■ Physical monitoring does not assure sterilization inside an individual pack or pouch of instruments.

## X.  DISINFECTION

Disinfection destroys most microorganisms by either physical or chemical agents. A disinfectant is used on environmental surfaces (counter tops) and other inanimate fixtures such as the dental unit and dental chair. Recognized methods of disinfection include the use of a chemical germicide registered with the EPA as a "hospital disinfectant." Chemical agents commonly employed in the dental office include glutaraldehydes, sodium hypochlorite, iodophors, and synthetic phenol compounds.

There are three levels of disinfection: low, intermediate, and high. The classification is based on the biocidal activity of the product.

- *Low-level disinfection* does not kill bacterial spores or the mycobacterium tuberculosis microorganism. Label may read "nontuberculocidal." Low-level disinfectants are used for general housekeeping procedures.
- **Intermediate-level disinfection** may be used on environmental surfaces. The label should indicate **tuberculocidal** (kills tubercle bacilli), and "hospital disinfectant" to qualify as an intermediate-level disinfectant.
- **High-level disinfection is sporicidal** (kills spores). Following manufacturers directions for contact time designates whether the disinfectant is used for disinfection or as a sterilant for items which cannot be sterilized under other approved methods of heat sterilization.

Manufacturer's directions should be followed for:

1. Appropriate dilutions of concentrated agents for environmental surface disinfection and instrument immersion
2. Preparation of instruments before immersion for sterilization
3. Proper exposure time for effective sterilization
4. Storage and handling specifications
5. Contraindications to certain metals and vinyl materials
6. Expiration dates

Adequate ventilation is required with the use of the disinfectant chemical agents because of possible eye irritation and toxicity from inhaled fumes.

## XI.  DENTAL LABORATORY DISINFECTION

Chemical disinfection agents may be used in the dental laboratory to disinfect contaminated impressions, dental prostheses, and wax bites. A chemical germicide with properties of an intermediate-level disinfectant is recommended. Communication between the dental

---

### Levels of Disinfection

Low-level disinfection is used for general housekeeping

Intermediate-level disinfection must display "tuberculocidal" and "hospital disinfectant" label

High-level disinfection kills spores

---

### When Using Disinfectants

Use manufacturer's recommended dilutions for concentrated agents

Clean instruments prior to immersion in high-level disinfectant

Follow proper exposure time cycles

Store and handle according to specifications

Do not use on certain metals or vinyl materials

Check expiration dates

Provide adequate ventilation

▶ laboratory and the dental office regarding the handling and **decontamination** (removal of contaminants) of dental materials is important.

All items that have been used in the mouth carry the potential for cross-contamination. Before items are sent to the laboratory, they must be thoroughly cleaned and free of blood and saliva. It is important to follow the manufacturer's directions for appropriate disinfection. If an impression or contaminated item which has not been disinfected is sent to the dental laboratory, it must be placed in a leakproof sealed bag and identified with a biohazard label.

To disinfect a dental impression prior to pouring, it is best to rinse the impression with tap water and then shake to remove excess water. The rinsed impression is then placed in a container or sealable plastic bag with the appropriate disinfecting solution for approximately 15 minutes. The dental impression is then rinsed again with tap water, shaken, and prepared for pouring. Contaminated impressions may also be sprayed with an appropriate disinfectant. *Following manufacturer's recommendations regarding which type of disinfectant agent to use on dental impression materials is required in order to prevent impression damage.*

## Summary

- A disinfectant is used on environmental surfaces (countertops) and other inanimate fixtures.
- Disinfection destroys most microorganisms by either physical or chemical agents.
- The three levels of disinfection are classified according to the biocidal activity of the product:

    Low-level disinfection is used for general housekeeping procedures.

    Intermediate-level disinfection must display a label indicating "tuberculocidal"/"hospital disinfectant."

    High-level disinfection is capable of killing spores.

- Following manufacturer's directions for contact time designates whether the disinfectant is used for disinfection or as a sterilant.
- Disinfectant chemical agents may cause eye irritation and toxicity from inhaled fumes. Adequate ventilation is required for use.
- Chemical disinfectants are used in the dental laboratory to disinfect contaminated impressions, dental prostheses, and wax bites.
- To prevent damage to impressions, follow manufacturer's recommendations for appropriate use of disinfectant agent.

## XII.    PRE-TREATMENT INFECTION CONTROL

Prepare the operatory by using approved cleaning agents on all environmental surfaces and inanimate objects before spraying with an intermediate-level disinfectant. A "spray-wipe-spray" technique is recommended. Then prepare the dental unit and chair with appropriate disposable barriers. Place plastic or foil covers on light handles and triplex syringe. Cover bracket table. Preset trays with bagged sterile instruments can be arranged in the operatory but left unopened until ready for use. At the beginning of each clinic day, the dental unit retraction valve water lines should be flushed by allowing water to discharge from the line for several minutes.

During the dental procedure, a separate disposable bag should be used to dispose of contaminated soiled materials such as bloody gauze or cotton rolls. A clean disposable bag for each patient should be attached close to the working area before treatment.

## XIII.  POST-TREATMENT INFECTION CONTROL

The auxiliary is required to use appropriate protective equipment during cleanup procedures. Heavy duty utility gloves are used when wiping down contaminated environmental surfaces and when handling soiled instruments. Countertops and dental unit surfaces that have become contaminated must be precleaned with an appropriate cleaning agent and disposable toweling before disinfecting with an EPA-registered intermediate-level disinfectant. *In order for the disinfectant to be effective, surfaces must be thoroughly cleaned of any debris or bioburden.*

All regulated medical waste is to be discarded in a separate plastic bag indicated for that purpose. Disposable needles and other sharp disposable items, such as scalpel blades, must be disposed of in an impermeable (puncture-resistant) container indicated for that specific purpose only. The auxiliary must take special precautions when handling sharp instruments for disposal to avoid accidental injuries with the infectious waste. A biohazard label is affixed to the designated container. Dental unit water lines must also be disinfected and flushed after treatment of each patient.

## XIV.  PREPARING DENTAL INSTRUMENTS FOR STERILIZATION

Soiled instrument trays are taken to the sterilization area for decontamination and preparation. Instrument sterilization involves the following five steps:

1. *Precleaning*—Instruments may be placed in holding solutions until ready to be placed in an ultrasonic unit. Placing instruments in a holding solution prevents blood and saliva from drying on the instruments.
2. *Cleaning*—The ultrasonic unit may be used to effectively remove debris from the instruments and minimize the potential of accidental injury from a contaminated instrument during cleanup procedures. To avoid airborne contamination, always keep the lid on the ultrasonic unit during operation. At the end of the ultrasonic cycle, instruments are thoroughly rinsed and dried.
3. *Packaging*—Instruments may be prepared in packs, tray cassettes, or assorted instrument pouches for sterilization. If instruments are wrapped in cloth, paper, or plastic, the material must be porous enough to allow penetration of the steam autoclave. Indicator tapes are

### Steps for Sterilizing Instruments

1. Preclean—holding solution
2. Clean—ultrasonic unit
3. Packaging—packs, trays, cassettes
4. Sterilization—heat sterilization
5. Storage—store in aseptic area

recommended for sealing the wrapped instrument kits to allow the operator to assess the effectiveness of the sterilization cycle. Indicator strips may also be placed inside the instrument bag.

4. *Sterilization*—Heat sterilization is recommended for all items that can withstand high temperatures. Autoclaving (steam under pressure), chemical vapor, dry heat, high-level disinfectant chemical immersion, and ethylene oxide are recognized methods of sterilization. Weekly biological monitoring is required for complete sterilization.

5. *Storage*—Asepsis must be adhered to after appropriate sterilization methods have been employed to prevent contamination of the sterile armamentarium and maintain the chain of sterility. Packaged instruments can be labeled and dated before storing in drawers that have been cleaned and disinfected. Instrument packs which become torn or punctured must be repackaged and resterilized.

# XV.   RADIATION ASEPSIS

Basic infection control procedures must be initiated when exposing and processing radiographs. Objects which have the potential for contamination must be covered by protective disposable barrier covers or disinfected. The x-ray tubehead, x-ray control panel, and exposure buttons, either wall-mounted or hand-held, can be potential vehicles for cross-contamination. Clear plastic barrier envelopes are also available for individual x-ray film packets. X-ray film-holding devices are considered semi-critical items. Approved sterilization methods for these items should be followed.

Processed x-ray films which are not in protective barrier envelopes are considered contaminated upon removal from the patient's mouth.

The contaminated exposed film packet is to be handled by the auxiliary with gloved hands only. Wipe with a paper towel to dry off excess saliva which may be on the surface of the film packet. (Contaminated exposed x-ray film packets may also be sprayed lightly with an intermediate-level surface disinfectant).

Carefully peel away the packet from the exposed x-ray film. Drop x-ray films into a clean paper cup without touching the outside of cup. Remove contaminated gloves, wash hands, and dry hands before feeding x-ray film into the processor.

# XVI.   MANAGEMENT OF OFFICE WASTE

Regulations regarding waste management disposal must be followed according to federal, state, and local requirements. Dental office waste should be handled as contaminated waste which has had contact with blood or other body secretions. If contaminated items would release blood when compressed or, if caked with dried blood or OPIM (other potentially infectious materials), the waste is consid-

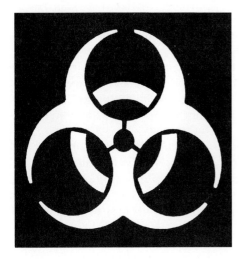

Figure 4–2.  Biohazard symbol.

ered regulated and should be disposed of according to local, state, and federal regulations.

Liquid waste, such as liquid collected from the high-velocity evacuation system, is contaminated with blood. Liquids contaminated with blood may be poured into a drain that is connected to a sanitary sewer system. Sink traps, suction traps, and evacuation lines should be flushed daily with water and a disinfectant solution.

Regulated medical waste also includes sharps and extracted teeth. Sharps are considered infectious because of the potential for becoming a contaminated vehicle capable of transmitting disease. Sharps must be placed in a puncture-resistant, leakproof container labeled with a biohazard symbol. Sharps containers are color-coded RED and should be autoclavable. If in-office autoclaving is taking place, the sterilizer should be spore tested when the filled sharps container is processed. Once processed, allow container to cool, then dispose of sealed sharps container according to local and state regulations. *Medical waste is also identified by using* **red** *leakproof plastic bags which indicate hazardous waste*. Biohazard stickers are recommended on all plastic disposal bags containing medical waste products (Fig. 4–2).

Dental offices may use approved waste haulers which meet EPA standards. Approved waste haulers use an identifying contractor number when removing regulated waste and generating the required paperwork indicating final disposal site of the waste.

## Summary

- Pre-treatment infection control requires pre-cleaning before spraying with an intermediate-level disinfectant.
- Flush dental unit retraction valve water lines for at least one minute prior to the beginning of each clinic day. Water lines are also flushed after treatment of each patient.
- Contaminated soiled materials such as bloody gauze or cotton rolls should be disposed of in a separate disposable bag.
- Heavy utility gloves are used to wipe down contaminated environmental surfaces and when handling soiled instruments.
- Surfaces must be clean of any debris or bioburden in order for a disinfectant to be effective.

- Disposable needles and other sharp disposable items must be disposed of in a puncture-resistant, leakproof container labeled with a biohazard symbol.
- The five steps required for instrument sterilization include: pre-cleaning, cleaning, packaging, sterilization, and storage.
- Processed x-ray films which are not in protective barrier envelopes are considered contaminated upon removal from the patient's mouth.
- Regulations regarding waste management disposal must be followed according to federal, state, and local requirements.
- Medical waste is identified by using red leakproof plastic bags which indicate hazardous waste.
- Dental offices may use approved waste haulers which meet EPA standards.

# Review Questions

1. Define the key terms listed at the beginning of this chapter.

2. List several methods of transmission of infectious microorganisms.

3. Identify and give examples of how cross-contamination can occur.

4. Explain why the concept of "Universal Precautions" should be practiced on all patients who receive dental treatment.

5. Discuss the importance of a complete medical and dental health history prior to the beginning of each treatment session.

6. What is the best protection for the dental health care worker against the hepatitis B virus?

7. When should personal protective equipment be used? Give examples of each of the following:

   disposable face mask

   disposable gloves

   protective eyewear

   face shield

   clinic jackets/lab coats

8. Identify how protective barrier techniques minimize the transmission of infectious microorganisms.

9. Discuss the importance of using an antimicrobial soap during handwashing.

10. List the five recognized methods of sterilization.

11. Identify how to determine which method of sterilization is appropriate for contaminated instruments. Your answer should include the following three categories:

   critical

   semicritical

   noncritical

12. List and describe the three methods of monitoring dental sterilizers as recommended by the CDC.

13. What results are interpreted from a positive biological indicator test?

14. Name the three levels of disinfection and indicate the biocidal activity of each.

15. Why is it important to follow the manufacturer's directions when using disinfectants?

16. Describe methods of disinfection in a dental laboratory setting. Include in your answer disinfection methods used during these procedures:

   before sending items to the lab

   prior to pouring a dental impression

17. Distinguish between pre-treatment infection control and post-treatment infection control.

18. List the five steps involved in preparing instruments for sterilization.

19. Discuss the use of protective disposable barrier covers with respect to x-ray equipment and related procedures.

20. Explain how contaminated x-ray films are to be handled and may be disinfected.

21. Differentiate between liquid waste, solid waste, and medical waste.

22. Describe the method used in disposing of sharps.

23. Why is it necessary to use biohazard symbols?

# Chairside Assisting

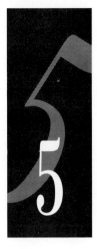

## Key Terms ◀

| | | |
|---|---|---|
| *CHARTING* | *MALOCCLUSION* | *PEDODONTICS* |
| *DENTAL IMPLANT* | *OBTURATION* | *PERIODONTICS* |
| *DENTAL PUBLIC HEALTH* | *ORAL–MAXILLOFACIAL SURGERY* | *POSTOPERATIVE INSTRUCTIONS* |
| *ENDODONTICS* | *ORTHODONTICS* | *PROSTHODONTICS* |
| *EDENTULOUS* | *OSSEOINTEGRATION* | *QUADRANT* |
| *FIXED PROSTHETIC APPLIANCE* | *ORAL PATHOLOGY* | *SEDATION* |

## I. INTRODUCTION

The role of the chairside dental assistant is expanding to include additional chairside duties and responsibilities. In some states, the chairside dental assistant with advanced training is allowed to perform extended dental functions under the direct supervision of a dentist. Updates in guidelines and procedures set by the office of Occupational Health and Safety Administration and the Centers for Disease Control have influenced and delegated additional responsibilities to the chairside dental assistant. The dental assistant must acknowledge and implement daily work practice controls in order to maintain office compliance under these regulatory agencies. In addition, the dental auxiliary must be trained in preventing and managing medical emergencies and be able to deal with all types of patients during routine clinical procedures.

The chairside dental assistant must have a working knowledge of all types of dental materials and be able to prepare, manipulate, and apply restorative and palliative materials for a variety of dental procedures. Coordinating dental assistants also participate in the practice of four-handed sitdown dentistry to increase office efficiency. This chapter will provide a synopsis of general chairside dental assisting principles and procedures including four-handed sitdown dentistry concepts and dental charting techniques. An overview of the recognized dental specialties is presented with additional review material for chairside assisting in orthodontics and oral maxillofacial surgery.

## II. ZONES OF OPERATING ACTIVITY

A basic principle of four-handed sitdown dentistry is proper positioning of the operator, assistant, patient, and equipment. The benefits of proper positioning include minimizing physical stress of the members of the operating team while maximizing visibility and patient comfort (Fig. 5–1).

To help visualize the positioning relationship in the operatory, the face of the clock can be superimposed on the properly posi-

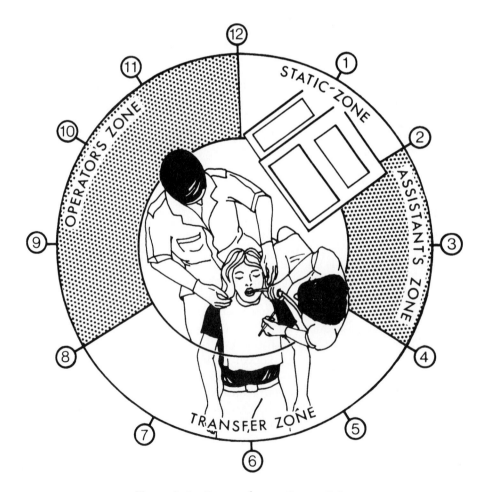

Figure 5–1. Zones of operating activity.

tip placement. The assistant holds the tip in his or her right hand (when working with a right-handed operator) with a reverse palm or thumb-to-nose grasp. When working on a posterior tooth, the tip should be positioned as close to the tooth as possible without injuring the soft tissue. The beveled tip should be held parallel with either the buccal or lingual surface of the tooth. While working on an anterior tooth, the tip should be placed opposite the surface of the tooth being treated, with the beveled tip parallel to and bisecting the incisal edges of the teeth. To avoid gagging, the tip should not be placed on the back of the tongue or soft palate. If it is placed too close to the water coolant of the handpiece, the water will be evacuated before it reaches the tooth. The tip should be positioned before the operator places the handpiece and mouth mirror.

A mouth mirror, oral evacuator tip, or both can be used to retract the cheeks and tongue. The operator using the mouth mirror and the assistant using the oral evacuator tip retracts the tissue closest to each. For example, a right-handed operator working in the lower right quadrant retracts the cheek and the assistant retracts the tongue.

## D. TRAY SETUPS

The use of prepared tray setups also decreases delaying factors. This system involves ensuring that trays are easily accessible and contain instruments and materials needed to perform given procedures in optimum positions.

Benefits of dental tray setups include adaptability to any procedure, ease of storage, minimization of interruptions to retrieve a forgotten instrument or material, and a decrease in time needed for preparing and cleaning operatories.

Trays are either plastic or metal. Plastic trays are lighter in weight and less expensive than metal trays. Moreover, they come in different colors and therefore can be color coded for different procedures. Disadvantages of plastic trays include the inability to be sterilized and decreased durability. Because metal trays can be autoclaved, they can be opened at the time of use to ensure asepsis. Disadvantages of their use include cost and the inability to be sterilized in small autoclaves.

The instruments and materials that are routinely placed on the trays are those that are used 90% of the time. The arrangement of instruments and materials on the tray is dependent on frequency of use. The more frequently an instrument or material is picked up and placed down, the more convenient and accessible it must be. For example, a tray setup used by an assistant working with a right-handed operator would have the hand instruments located on the left side of the trays. This placement is closest to where they will be used and in the most accessible part of the tray.

Hand instruments are placed vertically on an elevated mat to allow the assistant to see and grasp them easily. The tray must be kept orderly, and instruments are replaced in the same position from which they are taken.

## Summary

- Zones of operating activity for the right-handed operator are between 8 and 12 o'clock.
- The dental assistant's working zone is between 2 and 4 o'clock.

- Static zone contains less frequently used dental equipment.
- Transfer zone is between 4 and 8 o'clock.
- Eye level of the dental assistant should be 6 inches above that of the operator.
- Patient should be seated in a supine position for work in the maxillary arch.
- Patient should be seated between a 25-degree and 45-degree angle to the floor for work on the mandibular arch.
- Patients with respiratory or circulatory problems should be seated in an upright position.
- At the completion of a dental procedure, slowly return the patient to an upright position.
- Class I motions are used during most instrument transfers.
- Class II motions are used to transfer a double-handled instrument.
- Class V motions are fatiguing because they require refocusing of the eyes.
- Primary function of high-volume evacuation is to provide a working field free of saliva and debris.
- Bacterial aerosol is decreased by use of the high-volume evacuator.
- Oral evacuator tip may be used for retraction of the tongue and buccal mucosa.
- Oral evacuator tip should be positioned before the operator places the handpiece or mouth mirror.
- Preset trays decrease operatory prep time.
- Instruments and materials routinely used 90% of the time are placed on preset trays.

## III.    CHARTING

▶ **Charting** is the process of recording the present condition of the hard and soft tissues in the oral cavity. Symbols and abbreviations are used to minimize time and space on the chart. Reasons for accurate charting include facilitating treatment planning and permitting future comparisons of dental lesions. Dental charts also are used to identify persons involved in accidents and in other aspects of forensic dentistry. Accurate record keeping is critical when charting, and dental records may be legally used as evidence in a court of law involving malpractice suits.

Diagnostic tools used by the dental team to chart a patient's oral condition include radiographs, study models, health history, and clinical examination. The dentist using the diagnostic tools dictates the findings to the dental assistant, who records them on the patient's dental chart. Dental chart entries should be made in ink.

The location of each existing restoration and area of the oral cavity to be charted is identified in a standard manner. All tooth surfaces facing the midline are called mesial, and those away from the midline are termed distal. Surfaces of anterior teeth facing the lips are called labial, and those of posterior teeth facing the cheeks are termed buccal. All surfaces that face the tongue are called lingual. The biting edges of anterior teeth are called incisal, and the chewing surfaces of posterior teeth are called occlusal.

In addition to the symbols and abbreviations used to transcribe the existing conditions of the oral cavity, a tooth-identification sys-

---

### Tooth Charting Terminology

Mesial—tooth surfaces facing the mid-line

Distal—tooth surfaces facing away from the mid-line

Labial—anterior tooth surfaces facing the lips

Buccal—posterior tooth surfaces facing the cheeks

Lingual—tooth surfaces that face the tongue

Incisal—biting edges of anterior teeth

Occlusal—chewing surfaces of posterior teeth

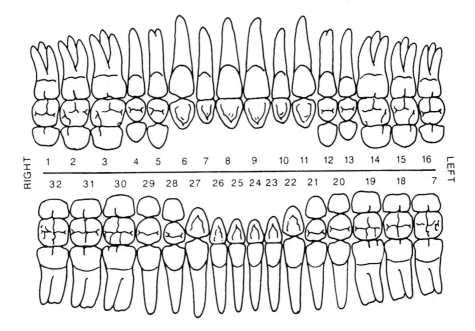

Figure 5–2. The adult dentition.

tem is used. Several tooth-identification systems can be implemented. The most popular include the Universal system, the Palmer system, and the International system.

## A.  THE UNIVERSAL SYSTEM

The Universal system identifies the adult dentition by numbers 1 through 32. Number 1 is the maxillary right third molar. The numbering proceeds around the maxillary arch to number 16, which is the maxillary left third molar. The mandibular left third molar is number 17, and the numbering again proceeds around the mandibular arch to the mandibular right third molar, which is designated number 32 (Fig. 5–2).

The deciduous dentition is identified by the letters A through T. The letter A is the maxillary right second primary molar, and the lettering proceeds around the maxillary arch to the letter J, which is the maxillary left second primary molar. The mandibular left second primary molar is lettered K, and the lettering proceeds around the mandibular arch to the mandibular right second primary molar, which is designated by the letter T (Fig. 5–3).

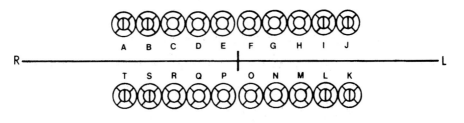

Figure 5–3. The deciduous dentition.

## B.  THE PALMER SYSTEM

The Palmer system divides the mouth into quadrants. Each quadrant in the adult dentition consists of the central incisor, numbered 1, to the third molar, numbered 8. In addition, horizontal and vertical lines are used and drawn to indicate each individual quadrant. For example, the maxillary right number 6⌋ and symbol represents the maxillary right first molar. The deciduous dentition also is divided into quadrants, with the teeth identified by letters A through E. For example, the maxillary right letter B⌋ and symbol represents the maxillary right lateral incisor.

## C.  THE INTERNATIONAL SYSTEM

The International system divides the adult and deciduous teeth into quadrants. The adult teeth in each quadrant are numbered 1 through 8, and the deciduous dentition is numbered 1 through 5. Another number placed before the tooth number indicates the quadrant in which the tooth is located. If the first number is 1, it represents the adult maxillary right quadrant, 2 is the adult maxillary left quadrant, 3 is the adult mandibular left quadrant, 4 is the adult mandibular right quadrant, 5 is the deciduous maxillary right quadrant, 6 is the deciduous maxillary left quadrant, 7 is the deciduous mandibular left quadrant, and 8 is the deciduous mandibular right quadrant. In this system, number 32 represents the adult mandibular left lateral incisor, and number 25 represents the maxillary left first molar.

The adult dentition is identified as follows.

## D.  PERIODONTAL CHARTING

A record of periodontal probing depths, recession, tooth mobility, bleeding points, suppuration, and root furcations, indications of periodontal disease activity, is charted using special symbols and abbreviations. These symbols are transferred directly onto the charting form to correspond with the exact location on the tooth. Six separate measurements are taken of each tooth to record periodontal pocket depths using a periodontal probe (Fig. 5–4).

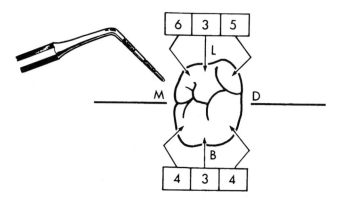

Figure 5–4.  Periodontal charting.

## Summary

- Charting is the process of recording present conditions of the hard and soft tissues in the oral cavity.
- Symbols and abbreviations are used for dental charting.
- Accurate charting is required for treatment planning and identification of accident victims.
- Dental records, including charting forms, may be used legally in a court of law.
- Radiographs and study models are utilized to chart a patient's oral condition.
- Tooth surfaces facing the mid-line are called mesial.
- Tooth surfaces facing away from the mid-line are called distal.
- Surfaces of anterior teeth facing the lips are termed labial.
- Surfaces of posterior teeth facing the cheeks are termed buccal.
- All surfaces that face the tongue are called lingual.
- Biting edges of anterior teeth are called incisal.
- Chewing surfaces of posterior teeth are called occlusal.
- Universal charting system identifies the adult dentition by numbers 1 through 32.
- Deciduous dentition is identified by the letters A through T.
- Palmer system divides the mouth into quadrants and uses vertical and horizontal lines to specify the quadrant.
- International identification system numbers each tooth in the adult quadrant 1 through 8.
- International system identifies each quadrant with the numbers 1 through 5 in the deciduous dentition.
- Six separate measurements are taken of each tooth to record periodontal pocket depths.
- Periodontal charting includes tooth mobility, bleeding points, root furcations, recession, and suppuration.

## IV. DENTAL SPECIALTIES

Dental specialties recognized by the dental profession include Dental Public Health, Endodontics, Oral Pathology, Oral and Maxillofacial Surgery, Orthodontics, Pedodontics, Periodontics, and Prosthodontics.

The dental specialist has advanced graduate training in a designated specialty field. More complex or difficult cases are often referred by the general dental practitioner to the dental specialist for treatment. A description of each specialty role follows.

### A. DENTAL PUBLIC HEALTH

Within the range of public health dentistry are the areas of community, municipal, state, and national dental health programs. The duties and responsibilities of dentists and auxiliaries depend on the scope of individual programs.

Many public health programs offer public education and prevention-oriented components, whereas others concentrate on research and direct patient care. The assistant's role in public health

---

**Recognized Dental Specialties**

1. Dental public health
2. Endodontics
3. Oral pathology
4. Oral and maxillofacial surgery
5. Orthodontics
6. Pedodontics
7. Periodontics
8. Prosthodontics

dentistry can vary greatly. In the direct provision of services, the assistant may perform tasks similar to those of an assistant in any private practice, whereas in public education, prevention, and research areas, he or she might assume complex roles involving the application of a variety of skills.

All clinical functions are regulated by state law, but auxiliaries in certain federal programs may be exempt from state restrictions. As laws regarding performance of functions vary from state to state, so too do the assistant's responsibilities. Some states permit assistants to perform expanded functions, tasks traditionally performed by dentists. These expanded functions include reversible tasks, such as placing orthodontic separators, placing and removing temporary restorations, and testing pulp vitality.

## B.   ENDODONTICS

▶ **Endodontics** is the specialty concerned with the treatment of pulpal and periapical diseases of the teeth. Some of the treatments involve pulp capping, pulpotomy, pulpectomy, instrumentation and obturation of infected root canals, and removal of diseased periapical tissues.

All diagnostic tests are designed to help the practitioner make a correct diagnosis. Percussion is checked by striking the crown of the tooth with the handle of an instrument to determine whether a tooth is sensitive. This is done in conjunction with the percussion of adjacent teeth in order to obtain subjective separation of symptoms by the patient. Palpation, the touching of suspected areas, can help determine whether swelling is present. The mobility test to determine the buccolingual range of movement, in conjunction with a radiograph, helps determine whether the remaining alveolar bone is sufficient to consider restoring the tooth. A radiograph is the most common diagnostic tool because it can help determine activity in the periapical areas of suspected teeth. Pulp testing by the use of heat, cold, or small amounts of an electric current through the application of an instrument called a vitalometer determine the vitality of a tooth.

Instrumenting the canal removes the infected pulp and prepares the canal for obturation, or filling. The instrumentation is accomplished by using reamers, broaches, and files. Reamers enlarge the canal slightly and are used to measure the length of the canal. Broaches are used to remove the affected nerve and any debris from the canal. Files are used to increase the diameter of the root canal so that it can be filled. All instrumentation is done using an irrigant, which serves to break down the soft tissue in the canal and lubricate the area. The preferred irrigant is sodium hypochlorite diluted with 1 to 2 parts water or hydrogen peroxide. The canals ▶ are dried with assorted paper points and medicated. **Obturation** or filling of the canal is done with gutta percha points and special endodontic condensers or spreaders. The gutta percha material can be compressed and condensed into the canal, sealing the apex. Once the procedure is completed and the apex of the canal is sealed, the tooth is ready to be fully restored to function.

## C.  ORAL PATHOLOGY

The specialty of **oral pathology** treats the abnormal conditions and ◀
diseases of the oral cavity and maxillofacial structures. A wide range
of pathologic conditions and manifestations may affect the dental patient as a result of developmental disturbances, such as cleft lip or
palate. Systemic dysfunctions and infectious diseases, such as AIDS,
may also cause oral lesions. Nutritional deficiencies and abnormal
growths or tumors are of concern to the oral pathologist.

Specialized tests, such as a biopsy that includes a minor surgical
procedure to remove a specimen of the suspicious lesion for further
study and analysis, require the expertise of an oral pathologist. Final
diagnosis of the abnormal lesion is made by the oral pathologist and
documented in a formal laboratory report to the referring general
practioner. Appropriate dental treatment for the patient may be conducted by the oral pathologist and oral surgeon in conjunction with
the general practioner. This specialty area is addressed in detail in
Chapter 1, Biomedical Science.

## D.  ORAL AND MAXILLOFACIAL SURGERY

◀

Oral surgery treatment ranges from simple exodontia to the most
complicated maxillofacial surgery.

All patients who are scheduled to receive treatment must undergo assessment of general physical condition (pulse, blood pressure, respiration rate, and body temperature) to determine whether
the patient can physically sustain the rigors of surgery. More complicated procedures require additional testing.

Preparation for oral surgery also includes treatment of pain and
anxiety through premedication. Administration of anesthesia is either
local or general, including conscious or unconscious **sedation.** ◀

During oral surgery, it is mandatory that aseptic techniques be followed to prohibit contamination of the operating field. The assistant
must be aware of the proper procedures for handling instruments. This
applies to the sterilization of instruments, as well as to their transfer.

The most common oral surgery procedure is the simple extraction. Teeth are removed with specifically designed forceps and elevators. Extractions of impacted teeth, retained roots, or alveolar bone
and dental implants are more complicated procedures.

Even more complicated procedures involve the treatment of
fractures of the mandible or maxilla and maxillofacial surgery, which
may include sectioning portions of the facial area to compensate for
abnormalities resulting from genetic or traumatic causes. In addition,
treatment of oral cancer is the responsibility of the oral surgeon.

After treatment, a patient may suffer from pain, postoperative
bleeding, and swelling. The patient must be protected against the
possibility of infection, which requires specific **postoperative in-** ◀
**structions,** including postoperative antibiotic therapy, if indicated.

## E.  ORTHODONTICS

**Orthodontics** is the study of the growth and development of the ◀
jaws and face. Also included are the position of teeth, influences on
development, and prevention and correction of malocclusions.

**Malocclusions** develop as a result of many factors. Face form, ◀

---

◀

**Oral and Maxillofacial Surgery Chairside Dental Assistant Must Be Able to Select and Prepare Dental Instruments for the Following Surgical Procedures**

Alveoplasty
Apicoectomy
Biopsy
Bone grafts
Dry socket treatment
Extractions
Fractures of maxilla/mandible
Frenectomy
General anesthesia
Hard tissue surgery
Hemisection
Hydroxylapatite augmentation
Impactions
Implants
Incision/drainage
IV sedation
Local anesthesia
Occlusal equilibration
Orthognathic surgery
Reconstructive surgery
Retrograde filling
Salivary gland surgery
Sinus lift
Skin graft
Soft tissue surgery
Splint removal
Suture placement/removal
Temporomandibular joint surgery

## Classification of Occlusion

Class I occlusion—mesiobuccal cusp of maxillary permanent first molar occludes in buccal groove of mandibular first molar

Class II occlusion—mandibular molars are in a distal relationship to the maxillary molars, lower jaw is retruded. Buccal groove of mandibular first molar is distal to the mesiobuccal cusp of the maxillary permanent first molar

Class II occlusion—mandible is anterior to its normal position. Buccal groove of mandibular first molar is mesial to the mesiobuccal cusp of the maxillary permanent first molar

## Orthodontic Chairside Dental Assistant Must Be Able to Select and Prepare Dental Instruments for the Following Orthodontic Procedures

Adapting extraoral headgear
Appliance construction
Archwire formation
Bonding procedures
Cementing procedures/removal
Cephalometric tracing
Diagnostic casts
Fluoride treatment
Impressions
Occlusal registrations
Oral prophylaxis
Orthodontic adjustments
Orthodontic emergencies
Photographs
Placement/removal archwires
Placement/removal bands
Placement/removal brackets
Placement/removal fixed appliances
Placement/removal ligatures
Placement/removal separators
Radiographs
Repair removal appliances
Splints

jaw relation, and the final position of the teeth depend greatly on heredity. Anomalies must be corrected to provide proper functioning in the mouth. Additional factors affecting growth of structure are diet, metabolism, and poor habits, such as thumbsucking, mouth breathing, and poor swallowing. The number and size of teeth are important and can determine the ability of a person to have a properly functioning mouth.

Three basic classifications of occlusion were developed by Dr. Edward Angle. Class I occlusion refers to maxillary and mandibular molars in correct relationship to one another. In a Class I relationship, the mesiobuccal cusp of the maxillary permanent first molar occludes in the buccal groove of the mandibular first molar.

In Class II occlusion, the lower molars are in a distal relationship to the maxillary molars, and the lower jaw is retruded, giving the appearance of protruding maxillary anterior teeth. Class II occlusion is further subdivided into two categories. Division I is characterized by V-shaped arches instead of U-shaped arches and by protrusion of the maxillary incisors. Division II of the classification is characterized by maxillary arches that are wider than normal and maxillary incisors that show a marked lingual inclination with an excessive overbite.

Class III occlusion is characterized by the mandible anterior to its normal position. Mandibular incisors may be in total crossbite in relationship to upper anterior teeth, and maxillary arches might be restricted in growth. The mandible protrudes prominently.

Diagnostic tools for classifying occlusion include clinical examination, health history, tooth relationships, and soft tissue appraisal. In addition, plaster study models, bite records, and cephalometric radiographs are necessary.

Resolution of occlusal problems is usually accomplished by tooth movement through application of measured forces in the desired direction. Teeth are either tipped or moved until they reach their new positions. Some teeth are more resistant than others. For example, molars are often more resistant than anterior teeth.

Orthodontic treatment can be either preventive or interceptive. Careful diagnosis and early treatment for relatively minor problems can minimize future patient discomfort and expense.

## F. PEDODONTICS

The area of dentistry concerned with the prevention, diagnosis, and treatment of children's dental problems is called **pedodontics.** This specialty recognizes that children present special problems to the dentist because of growth and behavioral factors. In addition, prevention and treatment of disease in the child permit identification of future problems in the adult.

Children must be given proper strategies to cope with subjective or objective fears of dental treatment.

Care of the pedodontic patient requires recognition that the purpose of treatment is not simply care of the primary dentition but management of the eruption and health of the permanent dentition as well. This involves treatment in all phases of dentistry. Particular attention is paid to prevention in an attempt to prevent caries through fluoride treatments and prophylactic operative procedures.

Thumbsucking is the most common oral habit exhibited by children. It is generally agreed that if this habit is not discontinued by the time the permanent teeth erupt, deleterious effects can occur. The severity of these effects is determined by the position of the finger in the mouth and the amount of force exerted. Other detrimental habits include lip sucking or biting, tongue thrusting, and mouth breathing.

The principles of general dentistry apply to the pedodontic patient, except that the situation is dynamic, since two sets of teeth are involved. It is therefore necessary to intercept and prevent the progress of dental disease by early and consistent treatment.

## G. PERIODONTICS

**Periodontics** is the specialty concerned with the hard and soft tissues that support the teeth. These tissues are the gingiva (free and attached), the attachment apparatus, and alveolar bone.

The primary cause of periodontal disease is bacteria in dental plaque. If plaque is not removed at least once every 24 hours, it begins to calcify and will eventually form calculus. Once the deposit reaches the calculus stage, it can no longer be removed by simple brushing.

Periodontal disease can be recognized with the help of radiographs and clinical examination. A full mouth series of radiographs shows the quantity and quality of alveolar bone loss. The approximate depth of each sulcus can be determined by use of a periodontal probe. Sulci depths in excess of 3 mm are considered a potential for periodontal disease, since the patient has reduced access for proper home care. The most important diagnostic tool, however, is visual inspection of the color, texture, and architecture of the gingiva as well as monitoring attachment loss over time.

Treatment of periodontal disease depends on the disease state. The most common treatment begins with scaling and root planing to remove calculus and plaque. Suggested treatment for disease that has progressed can include gingivectomy or gingivoplasty, periodontal flap surgery with ostectomy or osteoplasty, regenerative surgical therapy, or supportive periodontal therapy.

After scaling or root planing, if residual periodontal pockets or poorly formed gingiva remain with an absence of underlying bony defects but with a sufficient amount of attached gingiva, a gingivectomy or gingivoplasty may be performed.

Gingivectomy refers to removal of gingival tissue, and gingivoplasty indicates reshaping. These procedures are performed only if sufficient healthy gingival tissue remains after these surgeries.

If alveolar bone is involved, a periodontal flap is made to gain access to underlying osseous tissue. An ostectomy or osteoplasty, removal or reshaping of bone, can then be performed in order to return the oral cavity to an acceptable maintainable level of health.

Regenerative surgical therapy is similar to conventional periodontal surgical techniques but incorporates the use of new periodontal materials that can be placed next to the root surface of a periodontally involved tooth to promote regeneration of new attachment fibers of gingival tissues to the surface of the tooth root. Postoperative healing may require special oral hygiene instructions and should be explained to the patient thoroughly by the dental auxiliary before dismissal.

Surgical **dental implants** may be performed by the periodontist ◄

to replace missing teeth. A specially treated metal, usually titanium, is used to form the implant screw or cylinder. Endosteal implants are embedded into the bone and may require more than one visit to ▶ fully complete the dental procedure. Through the process of **osseointegration,** the metal titanium screw integrates directly to the underlying bone, creating a firm stable bond for the insertion of the prosthetic tooth. The dental auxiliary must follow strict surgical sterility procedures throughout the entire procedure to prevent cross-contamination of presterilized implant materials. Patient postoperative instructions and special oral hygiene home care instructions should be given before dismissing the implant patient.

## H.  PROSTHODONTICS

▶ The replacement of missing teeth in partially or fully **edentulous** ▶ mouths falls under the specialty area of **prosthodontics.** The task of replacement is accomplished with either fixed or removable prostheses.

▶ **1.  Fixed Prosthetic Appliances. Fixed prosthetic appliances** are used to replace missing teeth in the mouth when remaining teeth are sufficiently strong to support such appliances. A fixed prosthetic appliance, when put in place, cannot be removed. This appliance is used to restore normal mastication to keep remaining teeth from moving, as well as for esthetic purposes. Often this kind of appliance is a more satisfactory solution than a removable appliance.

In fabricating a fixed appliance, strong remaining teeth are used as abutments. The cemented bridge is attached to the abutments, which can be shaped to accept different types of retainers. Retainers can be full crowns, three-quarter crowns, onlays, or inlays. The retainers are connected to pontics, which are used to span the edentulous area. In the preferred construction, bridges have two fixed ends. Under very limited circumstances, however, bridges can have single fixed ends or cantilevers.

Frameworks are sets of retainers and pontics that are usually fabricated from precious or semiprecious metals. The esthetic replacement teeth are then fabricated and attached to the framework. These replacement teeth can be made from porcelain fused to the gold or acrylic veneers.

A bridge is designed to rely on satisfactory abutments identified by radiographs and study models. The teeth selected are prepared to accept the retainer. A temporary bridge is then fabricated to judge occlusion, esthetics, and the parallelism of abutments.

Final impressions are taken to make an accurate determination of abutment shape and the relationship of one abutment to another. Materials used for this impression may include hydrocolloids, rubber base, and polyether impression materials.

Final impressions are sent to the laboratory, where cast frameworks are fabricated. These frameworks are then returned to the practitioner to determine whether the fit is correct. An esthetic cover of acrylic or porcelain is usually applied, and the restoration is temporarily and, subsequently, permanently cemented in place.

**2.  Removable Prosthetic Appliances.** The number of missing teeth helps determine the size and complexity of the removable prosthetic appliance. If the mouth is completely edentulous, full dentures are required. If the remaining teeth can support the forces of mastication, a partial denture can be fabricated. Fabrications of full and of partial prosthetic appliances have some procedures in common, such as preliminary and final impressions and occlusal records. The impressions must be accurate representations of both hard and soft tissue structures. From these impressions, accurate trays for border molding and final impressions are fabricated. The final impression then represents both fixed and movable tissues.

Partial dentures rely on remaining teeth for retention and support. These teeth must be prepared to hold the components of a partial denture. Components of partial dentures include saddles, which lie on the edentulous ridges, clasps, which provide direct retention to the remaining teeth, and connectors, which connect saddles and clasps into a functioning partial denture. The success of a partial denture is a function of the design and interaction of the components (framework). By direct and indirect retention, the final prosthesis should be strong enough to resist the forces of occlusion. Once the framework is completed, bite registrations must be taken. Teeth can then be added to the framework to complete the partial denture.

Full dentures require accurate impressions for retention and comfort. An improperly fitted full denture can cause difficulty in speech, mastication, and retention. Retention depends on the surface area covered, peripheral seal, adhesion, and cohesion.

After final impressions are taken, the dentist takes accurate records of the bite (centric relation), face height (vertical dimension), face form, and tooth size in order to approximate normal structure. Materials used in making full dentures are acrylic and porcelain. Acrylics are used for both base construction and teeth, but porcelain is used only for the construction of teeth.

## Summary

- Public health dentistry includes community, municipal, state, and national dental programs.
- Endodontics is a specialty concerned with the treatment of pulpal and periapical diseases of the teeth.
- Diagnostic tests include percussion, palpation, mobility, vitalometer.
- Reamers enlarge the root canal.
- Files increase root diameter.
- Broaches remove nerve debris from the root canal.
- Obturation or filling of the canal is done with gutta percha.
- Oral pathology specializes in treatment of the abnormal conditions and diseases of the oral cavity and maxillofacial structures.
- Biopsy, a minor surgical procedure, is done to remove a specimen from the suspicious lesion.
- An assessment of general physical condition, including vitals, is required prior to oral surgery.
- Oral surgery requires treatment of pain and anxiety through anesthesia, either local or general.
- Sedation may be required during maxillofacial surgical procedures.
- Treatment of oral cancer is the responsibility of the oral surgeon.

- Post-operative instructions to the patient are required following surgical procedures.
- Orthodontics is the study of the growth and development of the jaw and face.
- Class I occlusion is the relationship of the mesiobuccal cusp of the maxillary permanent first molar when it occludes in the buccal groove of the mandibular first molar.
- Class II occlusion gives the appearance of protruding maxillary anterior teeth.
- Class II occlusion divisions refer to arch shape and form.
- Class III occlusion places the mandible in a prominent protruded position.
- Dentistry concerned with the prevention, diagnosis, and treatment of children's teeth is called pedodontics.
- Thumbsucking is the most common oral habit exhibited by children.
- Periodontics is the specialty concerned with the hard and soft tissues that support the teeth.
- The primary cause of periodontal disease is bacteria in dental plaque.
- Plaque will calcify and form into calculus if not removed.
- Gingivectomy refers to removal of gingival tissue, and gingivoplasty indicates reshaping.
- Surgical dental implants may be performed by the periodontist to replace missing teeth.
- Endosteal implants are embedded into the bone.
- Titanium is a specially treated metal used to form an implant screw or cylinder.
- Osseointegration integrates the implant directly into the underlying bone.
- Replacement of missing teeth in partially or fully edentulous mouths involves the specialty of prosthodontics.
- Fixed prosthetic appliances cannot be removed once cemented.
- Final impressions are sent to the dental laboratory where cast frameworks are fabricated.
- If the mouth is completely edentulous, full dentures are required.
- Partial dentures may be fabricated if the remaining teeth can support the forces of mastication.

# Review Questions

1. Discuss the basic principles of 4-handed sit-down dentistry.

2. What are the zones of operating activity for a right-handed operator?

3. What are the zones of operating activity for a left-handed operator?

4. Designate the zones of activity for the chairside dental assistant.

5. Identify the 5 classifications of motion.

6. In which zone do instrument transfers take place?

7. Describe the recommended method for seating a patient.

8. List the stages involved for instrument transfer.

9. Describe the transfer process and grasp of double-handled instruments and the anesthetic syringe.

10. What is the primary function of the high-volume oral evacuator?

11. Discuss several benefits for the use of prepared dental tray set-ups.

12. Explain the importance of accurate recordkeeping during dental charting procedures.

13. Define the following terms as they relate to dental charting:

    mesial-

    distal-labial-

buccal-

lingual-

incisal-

occlusal-

14. Identify the corresponding name of each tooth in the adult dentition utilizing the Universal system of charting.

15. Identify the corresponding name of each tooth in the deciduous dentition utilizing the Universal system of charting.

16. Describe the Palmer system of dental charting.

17. Describe the International system of dental charting.

18. How many measurements are required to record periodontal pocket depths per tooth?

19. What type of instrument is used to measure periodontal pocket depths?

20. List the eight (8) recognized specialties of the dental profession.

21. Describe several roles of the dental auxiliary employed in a dental public health setting.

22. Define the term obturation as it relates to the practice of endondontics.

23. Describe the diagnostic tests used to determine the vitality of a tooth.

24. What type of irrigant is commonly used to irrigate a root canal during endodontic treatment.

25. What is the purpose of a biopsy?

26. Why is it necessary to take and record the patient's vital signs prior to an oral surgery procedure?

27. Differentiate between general and local anesthesia.

28. Why is it necessary to sedate a dental patient undergoing extensive oral and maxillofacial surgery.

29. Describe why it is necessary to provide postoperative instructions to patients who have had oral surgery.

30. What can cause malocclusion?

31. Describe what is meant by Class I occlusion.

32. Discuss Class II occlusion and the corresponding divisions of this classification, Division I and Division II.

33. Describe Class III occlusion, including the facial profile.

34. What type of radiographs are taken to evaluate and diagnose orthodontic treatment?

35. Discuss the importance of patient management as it relates to children's dentistry.

36. What is the primary focus of children's dentistry?

37. List the hard and soft tissues of the periodontium.

38. What is the primary cause of periodontal disease?

39. Describe various treatment modalities for periodontal disease.

40. What is the difference between gingivectomy and gingivoplasty?

41. Discuss why oral hygiene instructions are important in promoting postoperative healing following periodontal surgery.

42. What type of metal is used for a dental implant cylinder?

43. Describe the process of osseointegration.

44. Discuss the importance of infection control during dental implant procedures.

45. What steps are involved in fabricating a fixed prosthesis?

46. Identify three types of final impression materials.

47. How is the dental laboratory technician used in the specialty of prosthodontics?

48. Describe two types of removable prosthetic appliances.

# Dental Radiology

## Key Terms ◀

| | | |
|---|---|---|
| *ALARA* | *EXPOSURE TIME* | *MILLIAMPERE (MA)* |
| *BISECTING* | *FILM BADGE* | *PERIAPICAL RADIOGRAPH* |
| *BITEWING* | *FOCAL FILM DISTANCE* | *PRIMARY RADIATION* |
| *COLLIMATION* | *FIXER* | *RADIOLUCENT* |
| *CONTRAST* | *INVERSE SQUARE LAW* | *RADIOPAQUE* |
| *DENSITY* | *KILOVOLT PEAK (KVP)* | *SECONDARY RADIATION* |

## I. INTRODUCTION

Through the diligent work of leaders in the scientific field and through advanced technology, x-ray films have become an important and sophisticated diagnostic tool in dentistry. Knowledge and an understanding of x-ray production are critical for the proper exposure of radiographs and the practice of radiation safety. Dental auxiliaries and dentists must be aware of potential radiation hazards in order to protect themselves and their patients. This chapter presents an overview of the principles of x-ray production, x-ray film processing techniques, methods of evaluation in identifying exposure errors, and occupational radiation safety.

## II. BASIC PRINCIPLES OF RADIOLOGY

Knowledge and understanding of basic principles of x-ray production are essential for the proper exposure of radiographs. X-rays belong to a group of radiations called electromagnetic radiations. Electromagnetic radiations or waves occur in different wavelengths and in both natural and manufactured forms. X-rays are manufactured and have short wavelengths. The short wavelength gives off high energy, which allows x-rays to travel through solid objects and penetrate dense tissues, including bone. Characteristic properties of x-rays include the following:

1. X-rays have no mass (weight) and are not perceptible to any of the senses.
2. X-rays travel in straight lines and cannot be seen in the visible light spectrum.
3. Like light, x-rays are capable of producing images on photographic film.
4. X-rays can ionize atoms or molecules.
5. X-rays are capable of causing biologic changes in the person exposed to them.
6. X-rays in high concentrated doses are used on human tissue to destroy areas of neoplastic cells (tumors) in the treatment of cancer.

The dental x-ray machine houses an x-ray tube where electrical energy is converted into beams of energy (x-rays) which can penetrate solid substances. There are three basic components necessary for the production of x-rays in an x-ray tube.

1. A cathode and tungsten filament to supply the electrons
2. A high voltage to accelerate or speed up the electrons
3. An anode, or target (focal spot), on which the electrons are focused and where they interact to generate x-rays

X-rays are produced when electrons strike the target. This produces a beam of x-rays that the operator directs toward the patient to record an image on the film (Fig. 6–1).

▶ **Primary radiation** refers to the main beam of x-ray energy emitted from the x-ray tubehead. The primary radiation records an image on the x-ray film.

▶ **Secondary radiation** occurs when primary radiation collides with matter. Scattered radiation is a form of secondary radiation and denotes x-ray beams that have traveled or have been deflected in all different directions. Scatter radiation is difficult to confine and may be scattered throughout the dental operatory.

All x-rays generated are not equal. Some have high energy, and others do not. Lower-energy rays, or those with longer wavelengths, are not useful because they have a lower penetration power and represent a radiation hazard. An aluminum disk 2 mm to 2.5 mm thick filters out the less penetrating rays before they leave the x-ray machine while letting the more penetrating rays through.

Since the film to be illuminated is approximately 1-1/4 x 1-5/8 inches, the spread, or divergency, of the x-ray beam must be controlled. Otherwise, areas peripheral to the targeted area would be exposed and would increase patient exposure. This process, called

---

### Characteristic Properties of X-rays

X-rays have no mass

X-rays are not perceptible to the senses

X-rays travel in straight lines

X-rays are not seen in the visible light spectrum

X-rays are capable of producing images on photographic film

X-rays can ionize atoms or molecules

X-rays are capable of causing biologic changes in the person exposed to radiation

X-rays in high concentrated doses are used on human tissue to destroy tumors in the treatment of cancer

---

### Basic Components for X-ray Production

Cathode and tungsten filament to supply electrons

High voltage to accelerate electrons

Anode or target on which electrons are focused and interact to generate x-rays

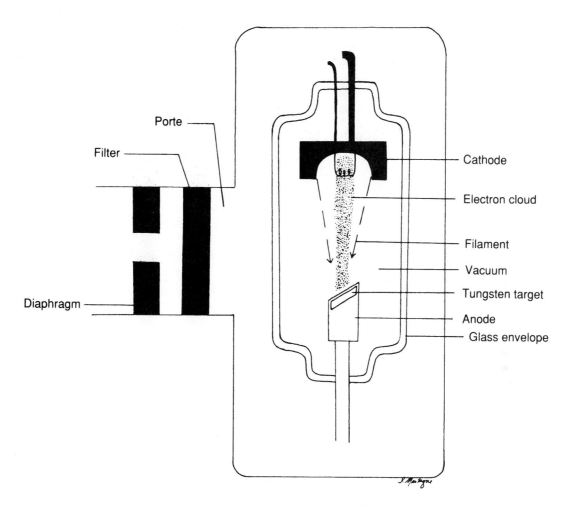

Figure 6–1. Diagram of x-ray head.

**collimation,** is accomplished by the use of a lead diaphragm which ◀ limits the size of the x-ray beam located within the x-ray tube.

Three parameters are controlled by the operator of an x-ray unit.

1. Quality (penetrating power) of the x-ray beam, expressed as **kilovolt peak (kVp)**
2. Quantity (number) of x-rays produced, expressed as **milliamperage (mA)**
3. Length of time the x-rays are produced, expressed as exposure time

The exposure time is usually the only parameter that is varied within a dental office. Suitable penetrating power for dental x-rays ranges from 50 kVp to 100 kVp and 5 mA to 15 mA.

◀ **X-ray Unit Parameters Controlled by the Operator**

◀

Quality—kilovolt peak (Kvp) penetrating power of the x-ray beam.
Quantity—milliamperage (mA) number of x-rays produced.
Exposure time—length of time x-rays are produced.

## Summary

- X-rays are capable of producing images on photographic film.
- The dental x-ray machine houses an x-ray tube where electrical energy is converted into beams of energy.
- X-rays are produced when electrons strike the target. The operator directs the x-ray beam that is produced towards the patient to record an image on film.

- Primary radiation refers to the main beam of x-ray energy emitted from the tubehead.
- Secondary radiation occurs when primary radiation collides with matter.
- Scattered radiation is a form of secondary radiation.
- Collimation limits the size of the x-ray beam.

## III.    RADIATION EFFECTS AND SAFETY

Radiation can be a useful tool for diagnosis and treatment planning in dentistry. Dental assistants must be aware of potential hazards associated with radiation in order to protect themselves and their patients.

Harmful effects of radiation occur in tissues as a direct or indirect result of exposure to x-rays. The degree to which radiation effects occur depends mainly on the total amount of x-ray exposure, the rate of exposure, and the type and number of cells irradiated. Cell sensitivity to radiation exposure varies with cell types and, in general, is directly proportional to their reproductive capacity. The cells most sensitive to radiation are young growing cells, reproductive cells, and blood-forming cells. Young growing cells are found in the pregnant dental patient, who should not have radiographs taken except in emergency situations.

The National Council on Radiation Protection has established specific radiation limits for operators of radiation equipment. The maximum permissible dose (MPD) for occupational exposure is 5 rem per year, or 0.1 rem per week. The dental auxiliary is responsible for assuring safe use of radiation in the dental office. Radiation safety includes three main elements:

1. Limitation of the radiation exposure
2. Limitation of the size of the primary radiation beam
3. Minimizing exposure to secondary or scatter radiation

Protective measures for radiation safety also involve both time and distance factors. The time factor represents the total history of radiation exposure. The operator must consider the patient's past history of radiation exposure, the number of films needed to obtain diagnostic information, the kVp, and the exposure time and film speed.

Distance factors affect the intensity of the x-ray beam. The **inverse square law** states that the intensity of the primary beam decreases in proportion to the square of the distance from the source. The dental auxiliary must understand this law in order to reduce his or her exposure to scatter, or secondary, radiation.

Radiation can produce both short-term and long-term effects. The term latent period is used to describe the time lapse from x-ray exposure until there is observable damage. Short-term effects, or acute effects of radiation, result from very high doses of radiation, as from a nuclear accident. Dental radiographs are not capable of such acute effects. Long-term, or chronic, effects occur years after exposure. Such long-term or chronic effects have been seen in operators who have held x-ray film in the patient's mouth during x-ray exposures. A dermatitis and subsequent development of cancerous lesions of the fingers is a result of this procedure. Other long-term effects of radiation exposure may include:

### Maximum Permissable Dose

MPD for occupational exposure is 5 rem per year or 0.1 rem per week

### Elements of Radiation Safety

Limitation of the radiation exposure
LImitation of the size of the primary radiation beam
Minimizing exposure to secondary or scatter radiation

1. Reddening of the skin
2. Hair loss
3. Split fingernails
4. Blindness
5. Sterility

Radiation protection guidelines recommend adoption of the concept of **"ALARA."** ALARA stands for "as low as reasonably ◄ achievable." The "ALARA" concept reminds the operator that every dose of radiation produces damage and should be kept to the minimum necessary to meet an appropriate diagnosis.

## A. RADIATION EXPOSURE TO THE PATIENT IS MINIMIZED BY THE FOLLOWING PROCEDURES:

1. Follow federal regulations and guidelines when purchasing x-ray units.
2. Periodically check x-ray machines for leakage.
3. Check machines to ensure that filters and collimators are placed properly.
4. Drape patients with leaded lap aprons and lead thyrocervical collars.
5. Use fast-speed film.
6. Employ lead-shielded open-ended cones/tubes, position indicator devices (PID), which reduce scattered radiation.
7. Avoid retakes.

## B. RADIATION EXPOSURE TO THE OPERATOR IS MINIMIZED BY THE FOLLOWING STEPS:

1. Stand at least 6 feet away, behind a lead shield, or both.
2. Do not hold the film for a patient during an exposure.
3. Use film holding devices for film placement.

No working area should be in the direct line of the x-ray machine. As a further precaution, all personnel should wear **film ◄ badges** that periodically monitor dosages. Workers who follow radiation safety measures should receive no unnecessary exposure to radiation.

## Summary

- Cells most sensitive to radiation are young growing cells, reproductive cells, and blood-forming cells.
- Young growing cells are found in the pregnant dental patient.
- Maximum permissible dose (MPD) for occupational exposure is 5 rem per year, or 0.1 rem per week.
- Protective measures for radiation safety involve both time and distance factors.
- Latent period is used to describe the time lapse from x-ray exposure until there is observable damage.
- The term ALARA stands for "as low as reasonably achievable."
- All personnel should wear film badges that periodically monitor dosages.

### To Minimize Radiation Exposure for the Patient:

Follow federal regulations and guidelines when purchasing x-ray units

Periodically check x-ray machines for leakage

Check machines to ensure that filters and collimators are placed properly

Drape patients with leaded lap aprons and lead thyrocervical collars

Use fast-speed film

Employ lead shielded open-ended cones/tubes and PIDs, which reduce scattered radiation

Avoid retakes

### To Minimize Radiation Exposure for the Operator:

Stand at least 6 feet away or behind a lead shield

Do not hold the film for a patient during an exposure

Use film holding devices for film placement

Film badges must be worn for monitoring dosages

Do not place working area in direct line of the x-ray machine

## IV.  RADIOGRAPHIC EXPOSURES

The dental auxiliary needs to understand that x-rays penetrate objects differently. This knowledge is used to adjust exposure factors to produce a high-quality radiograph. A high quality radiograph
▶ has good density. **Density** is described as the degree of blackness on the radiograph. Exposure factors affect the image on a radiograph.

The number of x-rays that hit the film determines the degree of blackening, or density, of the radiograph. Areas and structures that are denser, such as bone and metallic restorations, absorb more x-rays. Therefore, few x-rays reach the film, making the film appear
▶ **radiopaque** (white) in these areas. Structures and areas that are less
▶ dense, such as pulp chambers and sinus cavities, appear **radiolucent** (black) on radiographs.

The range of shades from white to black, including all shades
▶ of gray, is called **contrast.** The contrast of the radiograph is controlled by kilovoltage adjustment. Increasing the kilovoltage darkens the radiograph and decreases contrast. The density is increased slightly. Decreasing the contrast lightens the radiograph and produces more shades of gray and, therefore, the radiograph is more diagnostic.

Changes in milliamperage affect the amount of radiation produced. Increasing the milliamperage darkens the radiograph and increases the density. The contrast is slightly increased and produces fewer shades of gray. Density of radiographs is best controlled by adjusting the milliamperage.

Changes in exposure time affect density. Increasing the exposure time increases the density and darkens the radiograph. Conversely, decreasing the exposure time decreases density and lightens
▶ the radiograph. Milliamperage and **exposure time** work together to determine the amount of radiation produced.

It is important to minimize the degree of distortion in radiographs. Minimum distortion can be accomplished by meeting three criteria.

1. Only the most parallel rays strike the object and, subsequently, the film.
2. A minimum distance is maintained between the object and the film.
3. The object and the film are parallel to one another.

▶   These criteria, however, present problems. A lengthy **focal-film distance** (FFD) is necessary for the most parallel rays to reach the object.

The inverse-square law, which relates energy and distance, demonstrates that large FFDs require very high levels of energy. Therefore, an increased FFD necessitates increased exposure, resulting in increased radiation to the patient. The most commonly used FFDs in dentistry are 8, 12, and 16 inches.

Maintenance of a minimum distance between the object and the film (object–film distance) and parallelism between the object and the film are two criteria that compromise one another. The anatomy of intraoral structures prevents the film from being parallel to the object and, therefore, being as close as possible to the object (Fig. 6–2).

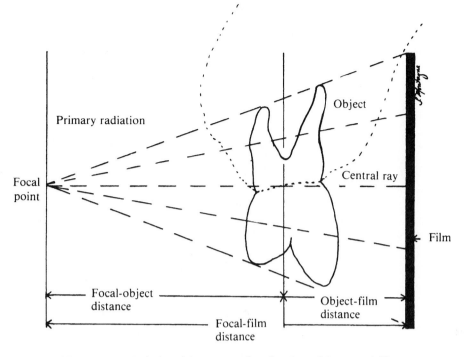

Primary radiation

Object

Focal point

Central ray

Film

Focal-object distance

Object-film distance

Focal-film distance

Figure 6–2. Relationship among focal point, object, and film.

## Summary

- Density is described as the degree of blackness on the radiograph.
- Radiopaque areas appear white on radiographs: for example, metallic restorations.
- Radiolucent areas appear black on radiographs: for example, tooth pulp chamber.
- The range of shades from white to black, including all shades of gray, is called contrast.
- Increasing kVp darkens the radiograph and decreases contrast.
- Decreasing contrast lightens the radiograph and produces more shades of gray.
- Density of radiographs is best controlled by adjusting the mA.
- Increasing mA darkens the radiograph and increases density.
- Increasing exposure time increases density and darkens radiographs.
- Decreasing exposure time decreases density and lightens radiographs.
- Most common focal-film distances (FFD) are 8, 12, and 16 inches.

## V.  THE FILM PACKET

The film packet must be moisture and light resistant, flexible, and easy to open in the darkroom. The film packet contains a waterproof outer covering, black paper, the film, and a piece of lead foil that absorbs any unused radiation. The foil backing also serves to reduce

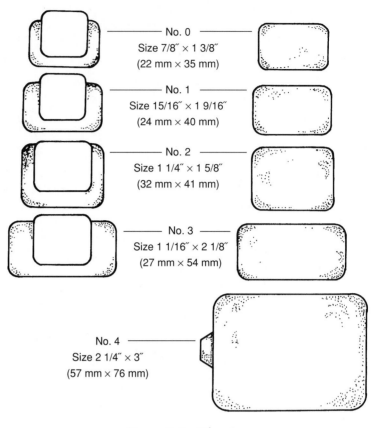

No. 0
Size 7/8″ × 1 3/8″
(22 mm × 35 mm)

No. 1
Size 15/16″ × 1 9/16″
(24 mm × 40 mm)

No. 2
Size 1 1/4″ × 1 5/8″
(32 mm × 41 mm)

No. 3
Size 1 1/16″ × 2 1/8″
(27 mm × 54 mm)

No. 4
Size 2 1/4″ × 3″
(57 mm × 76 mm)

Figure 6–3. Film size.

background scatter and thereby prevents film fogging. Double film packets, or duplicate film packets, contain two pieces of film. This allows for an exact duplicate set of films without exposing a patient a second time.

The film itself is composed of a silver halide emulsion, covered by gelatin, on a cellulose acetate film. The size of the silver halide crystals determines the film speed, or sensitivity. This film speed affects the amount of radiation and the length of time (milliamperes) required to produce an image on the film. Faster films have larger crystals and give poorer definition, or detail, on a film. Slower films, which have smaller crystals, give more detail and require more milliamperes.

Film speed is designated by the American National Standards Institute (ANSI) by letter groups A–F, with speed increasing incrementally with the alphabet. Fast films D–E are used most often in the dental office, combining fast film speed with an acceptable level of detail. Film size is manufactured in sizes 0 to 4 (Fig. 6–3).

Dental films should always be stored in a lead-lined container or compartment so that they are not exposed to scatter radiation, moisture contamination, heat, chemicals, or light.

Films that are outdated or affected by undesired radiation or light become fogged, which compromises their diagnostic value. Quality assurance measures can be implemented to avoid problems with x-ray film quality by periodic test film runs on selected film packets.

## VI.   TYPES OF INTRAORAL RADIOGRAPHS

**Periapical radiographs** provide information used to diagnose ◄ pathologic conditions of alveolar bone and teeth, including tumors, cysts, developmental abnormalities, and the presence of infection. Diagnostic periapical radiographs show the entire tooth or teeth from the incisal/occlusal edge to the apex (Fig. 6–4).

**Bite-wing** radiographs provide information useful in detecting ◄ the presence of interproximal caries and periodontal disease. Dimensional accuracy, clarity, image density, and contrast must be of excellent quality (Fig. 6–5).

Occlusal radiographs are frequently used to survey larger areas of the jaw (Table 6–1). The following is a list of indications for use (Figs. 6–6, 6–7):

1. To locate supernumerary teeth, impacted teeth, retained roots, foreign bodies, salivary gland calcifications, and other pathoses
2. To determine extent and shape of cystic, neoplastic, and infectious lesions
3. To locate and determine the type and extent of jaw fractures in tooth-bearing areas
4. To provide a means of radiographic examination for a patient who is unable to open the mouth wide enough for periapical radiographs
5. Record changes in size and shape of dental arches
6. To minimize the number of radiographs made during a pedodontic survey

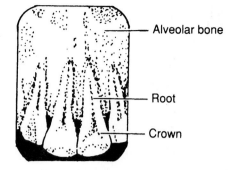

Figure 6–4. Periapical film.

### Indicators for Occlusal Radiographs

Locate supernumerary teeth
Locate jaw fractures
Record changes in size and shape of dental arches
Minimize number of x-rays during pedodontic survey
Determine shape and extent of neoplastic cysts
Detect salivary gland calcifications
Locate impacted teeth, retained roots, foreign bodies
Used for patients unable to open mouth wide enough for periapicals

TABLE 6–1. FEATURES OF OCCLUSAL FILMS

| ARCH | FILM PACKET PLACEMENT | DIRECTION OF CENTRAL RAY |
|---|---|---|
| Maxillary | On occlusal surfaces of maxillary teeth; patient bites down on film packet | Perpendicular to film packet; cone is 2–4 inches away from face; occlusal plane parallel to floor |
| Mandibular | On occlusal surfaces of mandibular teeth; patient bites down on film packet | Beneath mandible; perpendicular to film packet; cone is 2–4 inches away from face; inferior border of mandible aligned perpendicular to floor |

Interproximal caries

Figure 6–5. Bite-wing film.

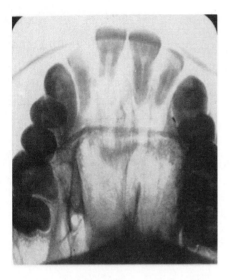

Figure 6–6. Maxillary occlusal radiograph. (Courtesy of Cerritos College Dental Assisting Department.)

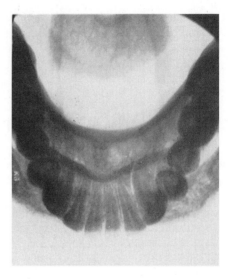

Figure 6–7. Mandibular occlusal radiograph. (Courtesy of Cerritos College Dental Assisting Department.)

## VII.  EXTRAORAL FILMS

Extraoral films are radiographs taken with the film outside the patient's mouth. The size of these films varies from 5 × 7 inches to 8 × 10 inches to 5 × 12 inches. These films are held in cassettes that perform the same function as the film packet. Most cassettes are metal, but lightweight plastic cassettes are used when taking a panoramic radiograph. Intensifying screens in the cassettes are used to intensify the radiation and, therefore, decrease the exposure time. Table 6–2 describes features of extraoral films (Figs. 6–8, 6–9, 6–10).

TABLE 6–2.  EXTRAORAL FILMS

| TYPE OF FILM | AREA VISUALIZED |
| --- | --- |
| Lateral skull | Whole skull pathologic survey |
| Anterior-posterior | Anterior-posterior plane of skull fracture survey |
| Water's view | Sinuses |
| Lateral oblique of mandible | One side of mandible, usually for third molar impaction |
| Temporomandibular (TMJ) | TMJ in various positions |
| Cephalometric (usually a lateral skull plate) | Identifies anthropometric landmarks essential to orthodontic diagnosis |

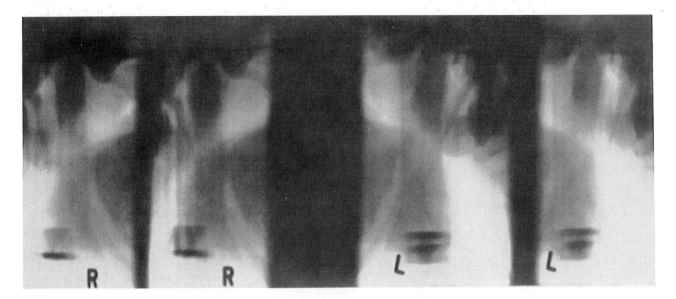

Figure 6–8. Extraoral film of temporomandibular joint. (Courtesy of Veterans Administration Medical Center, West Los Angeles.)

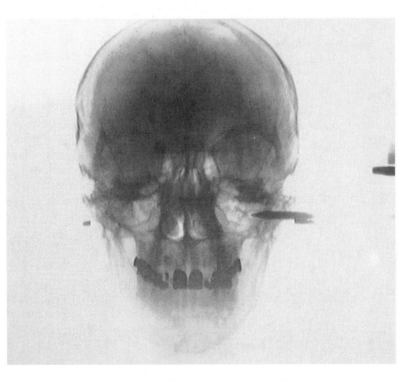

Figure 6–9. Cephalometric film, lateral view. (Courtesy of Veterans Administration Medical Center, West Los Angeles.)

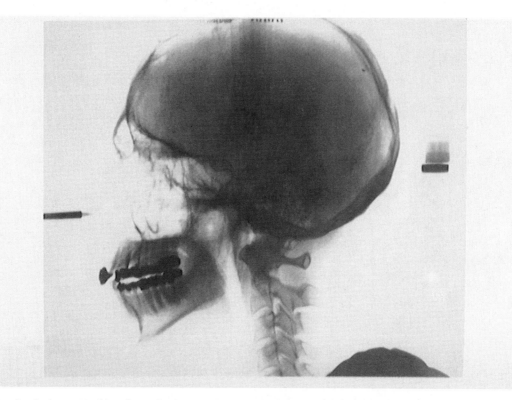

Figure 6–10. Cephalometric film, lateral view. (Courtesy of Veterans Administration Medical Center, West Los Angeles.)

## VIII.  PANORAMIC RADIOGRAPHY

Innovations in radiography have led to the ability to take a film of the complete upper and lower jaw simultaneously. This procedure is accomplished by using a panoramic x-ray unit. In essence, the patient's head is fixed and the x-ray tube and film focus and rotate around the patient's head. As a result, a continuous picture is produced on a single film. This type of film is excellent for evaluation of facial trauma (fractures), cysts, and tumors. It is also a very useful film to assess maxillary and mandibular dentition development and to evaluate the jawbones of the edentulous patient.

Some types of machines produce a film that displays a continuous image of the patient's jaws. In these types of units, the x-ray source rotates around the patient's face in a continuous elliptical arch (Fig. 6–11). Other machines are designed so that the x-ray source rotates halfway across the patient's face and stops while the patient's chair moves laterally to a second center of rotation, then continues to expose the other half of the patient's face. Because of the interruption in the exposure, a clear unexposed strip is created vertically down the center of the film (Fig. 6–12).

A panoramic radiograph of diagnostic quality includes the following features:

1. The condyles, inferior border of the mandible, and maxilla including zygomatic arches, sinuses, and lower portions of both orbits should be present on the film.

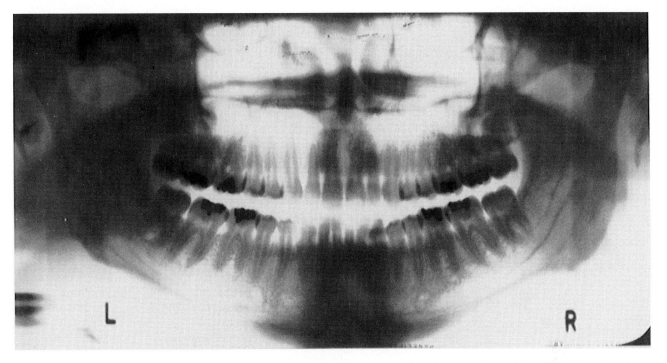

Figure 6–11. Panelipse film of adult dentition. (Courtesy of Veterans Administration Dental Service, West Los Angeles.)

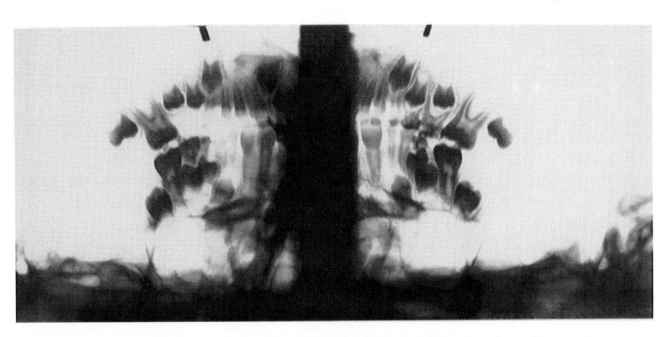

Figure 6–12. Panorex film of mixed dentition. (Courtesy of Cerritos College Dental Assisting Department.)

2. The occlusal plane should show a slight upward curve.
3. The teeth are the same size bilaterally without excessive overlap of interproximal contacts.
4. The anterior teeth are of normal size and are not distorted.
5. The condyles are approximately equal distance from the top of the film.
6. The contrast and density allow visualization of the soft tissue structures, such as the tongue, earlobes, and dental pulp tissue.

## A. ADVANTAGES AND DISADVANTAGES OF PANORAMIC RADIOGRAPHY

Advantages

1. Areas not seen on a routine full mouth series are shown.
2. Both upper and lower teeth are shown on one film.
3. Less patient cooperation is required.
4. Gagging is eliminated.
5. Less time is required.
6. The patient is exposed to a minimum amount of radiation.

Disadvantages

1. The radiograph is not as diagnostic as individual films for caries or bone height.
2. Images of teeth are enlarged or distorted.
3. There is overlapping of contacts in premolars and molars.

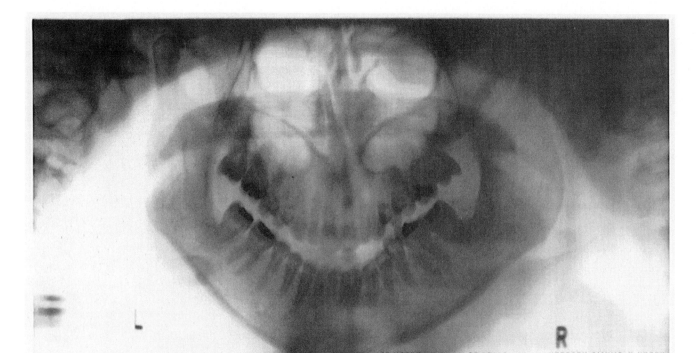

Figure 6–13. Chin tilted too far downward. (Courtesy of Veterans Administration Dental Service, West Los Angeles.)

4. Anterior teeth are difficult to see when they have pronounced inclinations.
5. Decreased sharpness and generalized haziness occur.

## B. POSITIONING ERRORS

Common positioning errors in panoramic radiography include improper chin tilt, noncentered patients, and tilting of the head to one side. Each error allows structures to appear distorted or to be projected off the film.

Chin titled too far downward (Fig. 6–13)

1. Mandibular symphysis is projected off the film.
2. Occlusal plane may exhibit an exaggerated curve.
3. Condyles may not be present on the film.
4. Anteriors may be distorted.
5. Excessive overlap of interproximal contacts exists.

Chin tilted too far upward (Fig. 6–14)

1. There is reverse occlusal plane curve.
2. Mandibular structures may appear narrower than normal, whereas maxilla structures appear widened, the palate appears thickened, and the film lacks bilateral image symmetry.

Head turned slightly

1. Images of structures on the side farther from the film appear wider and may be out of focus.
2. Superior portion of the condyle heads may be projected off the film.

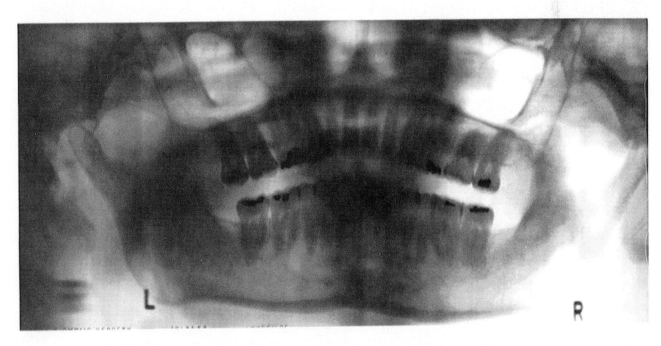

Figure 6–14.  Chin tilted too far upward. (Courtesy of Veterans Administration Dental Service, West Los Angeles.)

## Summary

■ X-ray film packets consist of a waterproof outer covering, black paper, film, and lead foil.
■ Lead foil in a film packet prevents film fogging and reduces background scatter radiation.
■ Size of silver halide crystals on film determines film speed and/ or sensitivity.
■ Film speed affects the amount of radiation and mA's required to produce an image on the film.
■ Film speed is designated by the "ANSI" by letter groups A–F.
■ Fast films D and E are used most often in the dental office.
■ Film size is manufactured in sizes 0 to 4.
■ Always store x-ray film in a lead-lined container.
■ Periodic test film runs are recommended to ensure x-ray film quality.
■ Bitewing radiographs survey larger areas of the jaw.
■ Extraoral films are held in metal cassettes.
■ Panoramic radiography is used to obtain an image of the upper and lower jaw.
■ Common positioning errors in panoramic radiography include improper chin tilt.

## IX. TECHNIQUES OF INTRAORAL RADIOGRAPHY

Two techniques are used to take a series of radiographic films: paralleling and bisecting the angle.

The paralleling technique is based on the principle that the object (tooth) and the film are parallel to one another, and the central x-ray beam is directed perpendicular to both (Fig. 6–15). Increased object–film distance results in loss of image detail, which is compensated for by using a long cone, (PID) position indicating device.

### A. ADVANTAGES AND DISADVANTAGES TO THE PARALLELING TECHNIQUE

Advantages

1. The image formed on the film will have dimensional accuracy.
2. Owing to minimum distortion, periodontal bone height can be diagnosed accurately.
3. On maxillary molar projection, there is little or no root superimposition.

Disadvantages

1. Intraoral film-holding devices must be used. These devices can be difficult to work with and uncomfortable for the patient.
2. Some patients have anatomic features, such as low palatal vaults, that prevent proper placement of film.

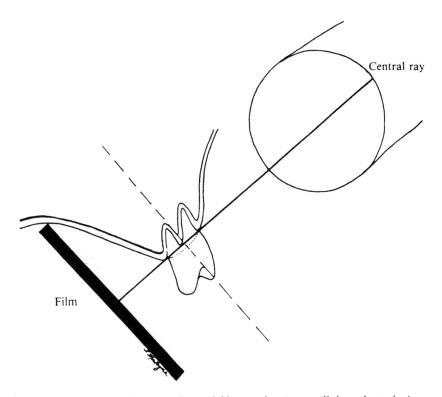

Figure 6–15.  Central ray, tooth, and film packet in parallel angle technique.

3. The use of a long cone (PID) position indicating device necessitates an increase in exposure time.

In the **bisecting** the angle technique, an imaginary line is iden-    ◀
tified that bisects the angle formed by the long axis of the tooth and
the film. The central x-ray beam is directed perpendicular to the
imaginary line. This technique uses a short cone (PID) position indicating device. (Fig. 6–16).

## B. ADVANTAGES AND DISADVANTAGES TO THE BISECTING THE ANGLE TECHNIQUE

Advantages

1. Decreased exposure time.
2. Less cumbersome film holder.
3. Anatomic features usually do not interfere with film placement.

Disadvantages

1. The image projected on the film is dimensionally distorted in varying degrees.
2. True alveolar bone height can be misinterpreted.

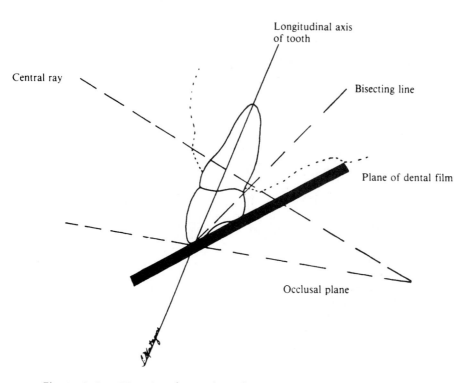

Longitudinal axis
of tooth

Central ray

Bisecting line

Plane of dental film

Occlusal plane

Figure 6–16.  Bisecting the angle technique of intraoral radiography.

3. The use of a short cone (PID) position indicating device results in divergent rays. Therefore, the image is not an optimum reproduction of the object.

# X.   STANDARD FULL SERIES RADIOGRAPH SURVEYS

A full mouth series of radiographs for an adult with a full complement of teeth is usually composed of at least 14 to 16 periapical films and 4 bitewing films (Fig. 6–17). Periapical films show the entire tooth and the supporting alveolar bone. They are used to diagnose bone and root pathologic conditions and to provide information on tooth formation and eruption.

Bitewing films show upper and lower teeth in occlusion. The full roots of the teeth are not visible on the film. Bitewing films are useful in identifying recurrent decay, proximal decay, the proximal gingival marginal fit of restorations, and periodontal bone loss. A two- or four-film survey may be taken. Two-film surveys are centered on the premolar/molar region. Four-film surveys include the premolars and molar views.

The following projections constitute a typical full series for a patient with a complete dentition:

Maxillary periapical projections

• Right and left central and lateral incisors
• Right and left canines
• Right and left premolars
• Right and left molars

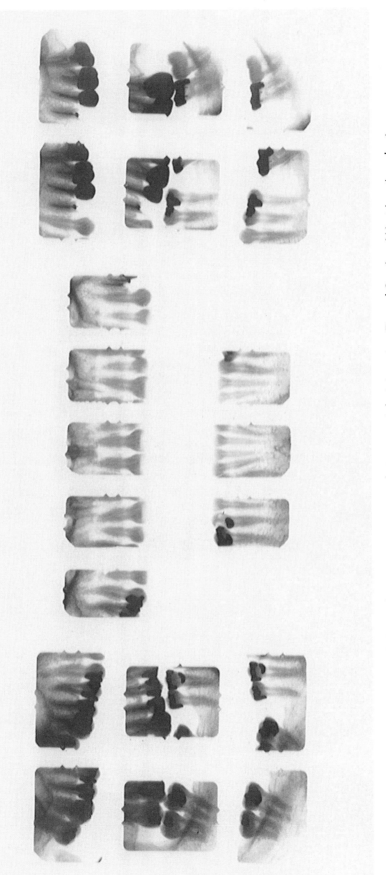

Figure 6–17. Adult full mouth survey. (Courtesy of Veterans Administration Dental Service, West Los Angeles.)

Mandibular periapical projections

- Right and left central and lateral incisors
- Right and left canines
- Right and left premolars
- Right and left molars

Bitewing projections

- Right and left premolars
- Right and left molars

A suggested sequence is as follows:

1. Maxillary right projections
2. Maxillary left projections
3. Bitewings (left, then right)
4. Mandibular right projections
5. Mandibular left projections

The pedodontic full mouth survey differs from the adult full mouth survey in the number of radiographs and the size of film packets used. The number of radiographs and the film size depend on the age of the child and the stage of dental development (Fig. 6–18).

The edentulous full mouth survey usually consists of 14 periapical films. Bite-wing films are not taken. Other modifications when taking an edentulous series include increasing the vertical angulation, decreasing the exposure time, and replacing the occlusal plane with the crest of the edentulous ridge. The edentulous survey is important in diagnosing pathologic conditions such as cysts and abscesses, and locating retained root tips and impacted teeth.

## XI.   RULES FOR EXPOSING RADIOGRAPHS

Regardless of whether the paralleling technique or bisecting the angle technique is used, certain procedures and rules must be followed.

1. Review patient's medical/dental history.
2. Seat the patient with head positioned so that the occlusal plane of the jaw being radiographed is parallel to the floor and the midsagittal plane is perpendicular to the floor.
3. Remove any eyeglasses or removable prosthetic appliances.
4. Drape the patient with a leaded lap apron that extends from the neck past the genital area and thyrocervical collar.
5. Turn the knob to the desired exposure time before placing the film in the patient's mouth. (A chart listing the desired exposure times for each area to be radiographed should be posted near the machine.)
6. After an exposure is made, remove the film from the patient's mouth. Dry the film and place it in a disposable cup.

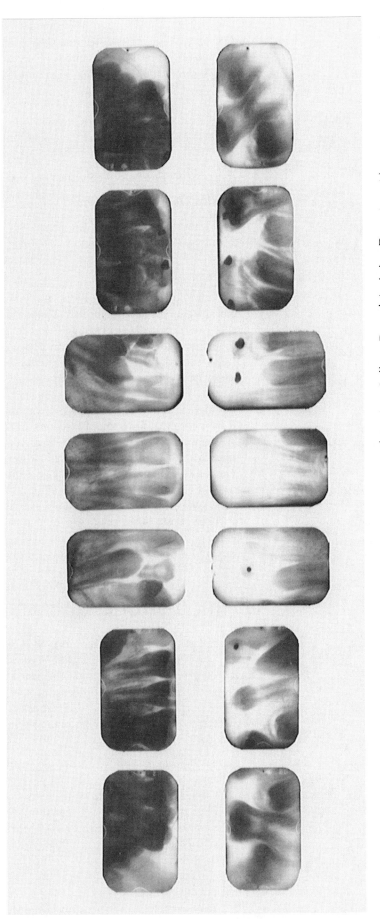

Figure 6–18. Pedodontic full mouth survey. (Courtesy of Cerritos College Dental Assisting Department.)

7. Never place films, exposed or unexposed, within an operatory where exposures are made.
8. Follow a definite order when taking a full series. Do not shift from area to area.
9. Use appropriate infection control techniques and protective barriers when exposing radiographs.
10. Use PIDs and aiming devices/film holders.

## A. *COMMON ERRORS IN EXPOSURE OF A FULL MOUTH SERIES OF RADIOGRAPHS*

Table 6–3 lists errors commonly made in the exposure of a full mouth series, as well as the reasons for these errors.

### Summary

- Paralleling technique is based on the principle that the tooth and film are parallel to one another and the central x-ray beam is directed perpendicular to both.
- Bisecting angle technique uses an imaginary line that bisects the angle formed by the long axis of the tooth and the film. The central x-ray beam is directed perpendicular to the imaginary line.
- Full mouth series of radiographs for an adult is composed of 14–16 periapical films and 4 bitewing films.
- An edentulous full mouth radiograph survey consists of 14 periapical films.
- Number of radiographs and film size depend on age of child and stage of dental development.
- When exposing radiographs, remove patient's eyeglasses and removable prosthetic appliances.
- Drape patients with leaded lap apron and thyrocervical collar.
- Use aiming devices/film holders to minimize retakes.

## XII. THE DEVELOPMENT PROCESS

A latent image exists on the film after it is exposed in the patient's mouth. The energized silver halide crystals must be processed through chemical reactions so that the latent image becomes a visible image. This developing process occurs in the darkroom. The darkroom is a separate room used specifically for processing exposed radiographs. The following components and requirements are essential:

1. No light leaks (films out of their holders are light sensitive)
2. Safelight (usually a 10-watt or 15-watt bulb with a red filter placed about 3 to 4 feet from the working surface)
3. Developing tank with three compartments
   a. Developer (usually on the right)
   b. Wash
   c. Fixer
4. Timing device
5. Thermometer (in developing solution)

TABLE 6–3.  ERRORS IN EXPOSURE OF FULL MOUTH SERIES
OF RADIOGRAPHS

| COMMON ERROR | REASONS |
| --- | --- |
| Elongation (most common error) | Too little vertical angulation; occlusal plane not parallel to floor; film not against tissue; poor film placement |
| Foreshortening | Too much vertical angulation; poor chair position |
| Cone cutting (clear film, curved line) | Beam not aimed at center of film |
| Film reversal or herringbone effect | Film placed in mouth backward |
| Film placement | Film not placed far enough in patient's mouth |
| Saggital plane orientation (occlusal surfaces appear because patient has leaned over; elongation and distortion) | Plane not perpendicular to floor |
| Overlapping | Incorrect horizontal angulation (central ray not perpendicular to center of film) |
| Crescent-shaped marks (black lines) | Overbent films; cracked emulsion |
| Light films (underexposed) (image not dense enough) | Incorrect milliamperes (too low) or time (too short); cone not approximating patient's face; incorrect focal film distance (FFD) |
| Dark films (overexposed) (image too dense) | Incorrect milliamperes (too low) or time (too long) |
| Double exposure | Film used twice |
| Fogged films | Exposure to radiation other than primary beam |
| Artifacts | Failure to remove prosthetic appliances, earrings, or eyeglasses |
| Clear films | Unexposed |
| Blurred image | Caution patient to avoid movement; adjust tube head and extension arm to prevent drifting |
| Poor contrast | Incorrect, kVp—too high; to correct, decrease kVp |

6. Rack on which to place films
7. Clean working surface
8. Sink (for cleaning tanks)
9. View box
10. Storage space

Before developing films, all solutions should be stirred to ensure that they are homogeneous and that the temperatures are equalized. Failure to maintain accurate records or to process films correctly will result in the need to retake radiographs, causing unnecessary radiation to the patient. A log should be kept noting dates of solution changes and daily recording of solution temperatures.

Appropriate measures must be followed for waste disposal of radiographic processing chemicals. Local, state, and federal regulatory agency requirements for the removal and disposal of hazardous waste must be followed. Offices may secure the services of a commercial waste disposal company for removal of the x-ray processing chemicals.

## A. FILM PROCESSING

Under the safelight conditions, each film should be carefully unwrapped and placed on the film rack. The development process for films is then accomplished in five steps.

1. *Developing*. The developing solution is a basic solution of Elon or metal hydroquinone that reduces the energized silver halide crystals to silver. The silver is precipitated on the film base and appears black (radiolucent). Since this precipitation process is dependent on the concentration and temperature of the development fluid, the radiograph is very sensitive to both the length of time in the developer and the temperature of the solution. The optimum time–temperature relationship is 4½ minutes at 68°F.

2. *Washing*. The developed film is then washed for approximately 20 to 30 seconds in running water. Washing stops the developing stage and removes any remaining developing solution that might contaminate the fixer.

3. *Fixing*. The **fixer** is an acidic solution that contains sodium thiosulfate and sodium sulfite, which removes the unexposed (or unenergized) silver halide crystals from the emulsion and preserves the picture. Potassium aluminum in the solution shrinks and hardens the film. Radiographs must be placed in the fixer for a minimum of 10 minutes, since inadequate fixation will cause the films to turn brown. Films may be removed from the fixer for inspection 1 minute after exposure, but should be replaced for 10 minutes to complete fixation.

4. *Washing*. Films must be placed in running water for at least 20 minutes. This final wash ensures removal of the fixing solution from the emulsion.

5. *Drying*. Films must be dried in a dust-free, clean area either by air drying or machine drying. Table 6–4 lists common errors made in the darkroom.

## B. AUTOMATIC PROCESSING

In recent years, automatic processing equipment that permits films to be carried on a series of rollers from solution to solution has become available. The appropriate time–temperature relationship is set, and dry films emerge in approximately 5 minutes. These machines save time, but they require periodic cleaning, and solutions must be changed regularly.

## C. DUPLICATING RADIOGRAPHS

Films which have been exposed and previously processed may be duplicated. Duplicating film has emulsion on one side only. To duplicate x-ray films:

TABLE 6–4. COMMON ERRORS IN THE DARKROOM

| ERROR | CAUSES |
|-------|--------|
| Record keeping | Racks not labeled |
| Fogged film | White light leak; faulty safelight |
| Underdeveloped film | Incorrect time (short) and temperature (cold); expended solutions (weak solutions) |
| Overdeveloped film | Incorrect time (long) and temperature (hot) |
| Developer cutoff (top of film is clear straight line) | Solutions too low |
| Clear films (emulsion washed away) | Films left in wash (running rinse water) for more than 24 hours |
| Stained film | Sloppy or dirty working surface |
| Scratched film | Racks hit; fingernails too long |
| Brown films | Films have not had adequate fixation |
| Torn emulsion | Films touching or overlapping while drying |
| Static marks (multiple black linear streaks) | Static electricity caused by friction when opening film packet |
| Lost films | Films not placed carefully in rack |

1. Enter darkroom and turn on safelight.
2. Place films on duplicator machine glass.
3. Place duplicating film emulsion side down on top of the radiographs.
4. Turn on duplicating machine light according to manufacturer's recommendations.
5. Remove duplicating film from duplicating machine and process in wet tanks or automatic processor. (Darkroom safelight remains on during this process).

# XIII.   STEPS FOR MOUNTING RADIOGRAPHS

1. Separate the films into three piles.
   a. *Anterior periapicals.* The teeth are shown on the film vertically (up and down).
   b. *Posterior periapicals.* The teeth are shown on the film horizontally (across).
   c. *Bitewings.* The crowns of both the upper and lower teeth are shown on the film (the roots are not visible).
2. View the anterior films with the dot facing outward (labial mounting). Separate the maxillary films from the mandibular films. They can be identified by referring to anatomic landmarks (Tables 6–5 and 6–6).
3. Mount the anterior periapical films. The incisal edges of the maxillary anteriors are to be facing downward. The incisal edges of the mandibular anteriors are to be facing upward. (This is the same position as the teeth in the mount.)
4. View the posterior films with the dot facing outward. Separate the mandibular films from the maxillary films.
5. Mount the posterior periapicals. The occlusal surfaces of the maxillary teeth are to be facing downward. The oc-

TABLE 6–5. RADIOLUCENT ANATOMIC LANDMARKS

| AREA | LANDMARKS |
|---|---|
| Mandibular molar | 1. Mandibular canal (inferior alveolar canal)<br>2. Mandibular foramen |
| Mandibular premolar | 1. Mental foramen<br>2. Mandibular canal |
| Mandibular cuspid | 1. Mental foramen (position varies) |
| Mandibular incisor | 1. Lingual foramen |
| Maxillary premolar | 1. Anterior portion of maxillary sinus |
| Maxillary cuspid | 1. Nasal fossae<br>2. Maxillary sinus |
| Maxillary incisor | 1. Incisive foramen and portion of incisive canal<br>2. Median palatine suture<br>3. Nasal fossae<br>4. Outline of nasal shadow |

clusal surfaces of the mandibular teeth are to be facing upward.

6. View the bitewing films with the dot facing outward.
7. Mount the bitewings. The bitewings should match with the crowns of the periapical films directly above.
8. Check the mounted radiographs to be sure:
   a. All dots are facing same direction.
   b. All incisal and occlusal surfaces are facing in the proper direction.

TABLE 6–6. RADIOPAQUE ANATOMIC LANDMARKS

| AREA | LANDMARKS |
|---|---|
| Mandibular molar | 1. Anterior border of ramus<br>2. External oblique line<br>3. Mylohyoid line—internal oblique<br>4. Impacted third molar |
| Mandibular premolar | 1. Inferior border of mandible<br>2. Mylohyoid line or ridge<br>3. Mandibular tori |
| Mandibular cuspid | 1. Mental process<br>2. Inferior border of mandible |
| Mandibular incisor | 1. Genial spine or tubercle<br>2. Mental prominence<br>3. Inferior border of mandible<br>4. Mental symphysis |
| Maxillary molar | 1. Coronoid process<br>2. Pterygoid hamulus<br>3. Zygomatic arch<br>4. Maxillary tuberosity<br>5. Outline of maxillary sinus |
| Maxillary premolar | 1. U-shaped zygomatic process<br>2. Floor of nasal cavity<br>3. Outline of maxillary sinus |
| Maxillary cuspid | 1. Inverted Y-formation of maxillary sinus |
| Maxillary incisor | 1. Median nasal septum<br>2. Outline of soft tissue of nose |

    c. Radiographs on right side of mount are matching (restorations, missing teeth, impactions, and so on).

    d. Radiographs on left side of mount are matching.

## A. LANDMARKS TO FACILITATE MOUNTING

Anatomic landmarks are those normal structures and areas that appear in a routine series of radiographs. These structures will not appear, however, with the same clarity for all patients. The terms radiolucent and radiopaque refer to the penetration ability of x-rays. The term radiolucent describes the dark areas that appear on the radiograph. Tissues such as oral mucosa, pulp, and gingiva provide little or no resistance and x-rays can easily penetrate these thin or less dense objects. This is in contrast to the very light areas on the film. Structures that are very thick or dense, such as amalgam restorations, enamel, and bone, absorb most x-rays and do not permit them to reach the film. These structures are termed radiopaque and appear white. Tables 6–5 and 6–6 list radiopaque and radiolucent anatomic landmarks that can be identified on a series of radiographs.

## B. ADDITIONAL GUIDELINES TO FACILITATE MOUNTING

1. The slight curve upward from the cuspid area toward the molar area, formed by the occlusal (biting) surfaces of the teeth
2. The upward curve of bone at the end of the mandibular arch
3. The appearance of the area behind the maxillary molar (shadows formed) as compared with the appearance of the area behind the mandibular molars (definite shape of the mandible)
4. The root difference between maxillary and mandibular teeth
5. Root tips that usually curve toward the distal
6. The differing bone densities in the mandibular and maxillary arches
7. The differences in size of anterior teeth (mandibular anterior teeth are smaller than the maxillary anterior teeth)
8. The darkened area (maxillary sinus is radiolucent) usually visible above and between the roots of the maxillary premolars and molar areas
9. The white lines (floor and walls of the cavities and sinuses) visible on the maxillary arch
10. Maxillary first premolars usually have two roots, whereas mandibular premolars have one root. Mandibular first and second molars usually have two divergent curved roots with bone clearly visible between them. This is particularly true of the first molar. Maxillary molars have three roots, two buccal and one palatal. The large palatal root obscures the intraradicular bone.

Mounted radiographs are read by the dentist for interpretation and diagnosis on an illuminated viewbox. Once radiographs have been read, the mounted films are placed in a protective envelope and filed in the patient's dental chart. Protection of the mounted x-rays from scratching is important. All x-ray films taken must be filed and stored along with the patient's permanent dental record for legal purposes.

# XIV. INFECTION CONTROL AND RADIOGRAPHS

Exposing, processing, and mounting dental radiographs are considered a potential source for disease transmission. Infection control procedures should always be considered and followed thoroughly. The tube head and exposure control switch must be protected with barrier covers. Personal protective equipment must be worn during patient contact. Individual film packets are available in clear plastic barrier envelopes to facilitate infection control protocols in the darkroom. Film holding instruments must always be sterilized if they are not disposable.

After exposing intraoral radiographs, wipe the film with a paper towel or gauze to remove saliva. A light spray of disinfectant on the contaminated x-ray packet may also be used as long as there is no moisture contamination. Place the exposed film in a disposable paper cup for processing.

In the darkroom, carefully unwrap the film packets, spill the untouched film on an uncontaminated flat surface, and dispose of the wrappings in a waste receptacle. When all of the films have been unwrapped, remove and discard gloves in the waste receptacle and deposit the film in the automatic processor or place on film racks. If the automatic film processor has a daylight loader, the constant contamination of the fabric light shield must be recognized. When gloved, contaminated hands are inserted through the elastic light shield, the fabric is repeatedly soiled, and there is no practical way to disinfect this material. The following procedure is suggested:

1. Place the exposed film in a paper cup and remove soiled gloves.
2. Use clean gloved hands to place cup inside the daylight loader and close lid.
3. Pass clean, gloved hands through the light shield to unwrap the film.
4. Drop the film onto the uncontaminated surface inside the loader.
5. Place the soiled film wrapping in the cup.
6. Remove soiled gloves and place them in the paper cup.
7. Place film into the chute for developing.

Surfaces in the darkroom that may become contaminated must be cleaned and disinfected with an approved EPA intermediate-level surface disinfectant agent.

## Summary

- The darkroom is used for processing exposed radiographs.
- Before developing films, stir processing solutions and check temperatures.
- A log is kept to monitor dates of solution changes and solution temperatures.

- Appropriate measures must be followed for waste disposal of radiographic processing chemicals.
- Developing solutions reduce the energized silver halide crystals to silver.
- Films are placed in running water (wash) for 20–30 seconds to remove any remaining developing solution.
- Fixer removes the unexposed silver halide crystals from the emulsion and preserves the picture.
- Radiographs must be placed in the fixer for a minimum of 10 minutes.
- After films are fixed, return to final wash tank for at least 20 minutes.
- Films must be dried in a dust-free, clean area.
- X-ray films which have been exposed may be duplicated.
- To mount radiographs correctly, refer to anatomic landmarks.
- Incisal edges of maxillary anteriors are mounted facing downward.
- Incisal edges of mandibular anteriors are mounted facing upward.
- Occlusal edges of maxillary molars are mounted facing downward.
- Occlusal edges of mandibular molars are mounted facing upward.
- Mounted bitewings should match with the crowns of the periapical films.
- Mounted radiographs are read on an illuminated x-ray viewbox.
- All x-ray films must be filed and stored along with the patient's permanent dental record for legal purposes.
- Infection control practices must be implemented when exposing and processing radiographs.

# Review Questions

1. Define the key terms listed at the beginning of this chapter.

2. Describe the principles of x-ray production.

3. List the characteristic properties of x-rays.

4. Explain the biologic dangers associated with ionizing radiation.

5. What are the 3 basic components found in an x-ray tube?

6. What is meant by the term scattered radiation?

7. Discuss the process of collimation.

8. List 3 parameters controlled by the operator of an x-ray unit.

9. Describe what is meant by MPD.

10. Explain the inverse-square law and how it relates to radiation safety.

11. List examples of the long-term effects of radiation exposure on the human body.

12. Discuss the "ALARA" concept.

13. Identify several factors which may minimize radiation exposure to the patient.

14. Identify factors which may minimize occupational radiation exposure for the operator.

15. Describe adjustments in kVp which influence film contrast.

16. Describe how mA affects radiographic density.

17. How can radiographic distortion be accomplished?

18. Identify the components of an x-ray film packet.

19. List the sizes of x-ray film.

20. Describe the various types of intraoral radiographs.

21. Why are extraoral radiographs required?

22. Discuss how the panoramic radiograph is taken.

23. List the diagnostic features of a panoramic radiograph.

24. Identify common positioning errors which can occur when taking a panoramic radiograph.

25. Define the following two exposure techniques for producing diagnostic x-rays.
    • paralleling exposure technique-
    • bisecting angle technique-

26. Differentiate between the advantages and disadvantages of the paralleling technique and bisecting technique.

27. How many films are there in an adult full mouth radiographic series?

28. Describe why bitewing x-ray films are taken.

29. List the projections and identify the views of the teeth which are visible in an adult full mouth series.

30. Why are films taken on an edentulous patient?

31. List 10 rules which should be followed when exposing dental x-rays.

32. Identify the chemical components used in developing and processing exposed x-ray films.

33. Describe the processing equipment found in a typical darkroom.

34. Discuss the appropriate method for waste disposal of radiographic processing chemicals.

35. List the five steps required to safely process exposed x-ray films. Your answer should include manual and automatic processing techniques.

36. Describe the steps for duplicating radiographs.

37. Identify the steps for mounting radiographs.

38. Identify how landmarks can facilitate mounting radiographs.

39. Describe the rationale for infection control procedures during exposing and processing x-ray procedures.

# Dental Materials

## Key Terms ◀

| | | |
|---|---|---|
| *Acid Etch* | *Exothermic* | *Monomer* |
| *Alginate* | *Gypsum* | *Polymer* |
| *Composite* | *Imbibition* | *Polymerization* |
| *Elastomers* | *Light Cure* | *Syneresis* |
| *Endothermic* | *Mercury Toxicity* | *Trituration* |

## I. INTRODUCTION

The science of dental materials includes a wide range of natural and synthetic substances and products used in the delivery of oral health care. Auxiliaries play an essential role in the preparation, manipulation, and application of dental materials in the dental office. Consequently, a thorough understanding of the physical and biologic properties of dental materials is necessary for the dental auxiliary in order to perform effectively and accurately when preparing, manipulating, and applying dental materials. This chapter provides a synopsis of dental restorative materials, dental cements, gypsum products, impression materials, endodontic, and sedative dental materials.

| Matter Exists in Three States |
| --- |
| Solid<br>Liquid<br>Gas |

## II.  PROPERTIES OF MATTER

The science of dental materials requires a basic understanding of the properties of matter. All dental materials are made up of atomic matter that directly affects the chemical and physical working properties of the material. Matter exists in three different states: solid, liquid, and gas. By altering temperature and pressure, most materials can be changed to any of the three states. Temperature is a measure of the intensity of heat. The amount of heat evolved or absorbed during a chemical reaction is called the heat of reaction. If heat is evolved, or given off, the reaction is described as **exothermic.** If heat is absorbed, the reaction is **endothermic.** The setting of dental stone and acrylic exhibits exothermic reactions. Caution must be exercised when using these materials intraorally to avoid damaging the pulpal tissues and oral mucosa.

Heat is measured in either Fahrenheit or Celsius degrees, and temperature expressed by one system can be easily converted to the other.

To convert degrees Fahrenheit to degrees Celsius, the following formula is used:

$$°C = 5/9 \ (°F - 32)$$

To convert degrees Celsius to degrees Fahrenheit, the following formula is used:

$$°F = 9/5 \ (°C + 32)$$

## III.  GYPSUM PRODUCTS: PLASTER AND STONE

**Gypsum** products are used in dentistry to form casts and dies that are positive reproductions of patients' hard and soft oral tissues. These materials can also be used intraorally as impression materials for taking full denture impressions or soldering registrations for casting. Intraoral use of gypsum products is diminishing, however, since other materials can give equal accuracy and detail and are easier to use intraorally.

Plasters and stones are made by grinding gypsum under high temperatures (230–250°F) to drive off part of the water of crystallization. This process is called calcination. The main constituent of all plasters or stones is calcium sulfate hemihydrate. The degree of refinement of the calcium sulfate hemihydrate is contingent on whether plaster or stone is desired. Particles in plaster are more irregular and spongy, whereas stone has more dense particles in more crystalline forms. The difference in particle shape between plasters and stones reflects the difference in properties. Plasters are not as strong as stones, although both are easy to manipulate.

Stone can be further classified into class I and II stones. Class I stone contains more regular particles and is used mainly for pouring casts. Study casts are used to record conditions of the mouth and provide valuable treatment planning information for the dentist (Table 7–1). Class II stone, also known as improved stone (high-strength stone), contains a greater number of random-shaped particles and, as a result, is a harder material. Improved stone is used primarily to make dies.

Gypsum products produce an exothermic reaction (heat is released). The amount of water mixed with the plaster or stone is very important and is expressed as the water to powder (w/p) ratio. For example, the more water added, the longer the setting time and the

TABLE 7–1. VALUE OF DIAGNOSTIC CAST STUDY MODELS

1. Assist in diagnosis and treatment planning
2. Patient education
3. Record treatment and growth
4. Record tooth form, position, occlusion, and anatomy of restorations
5. Serve as "Before" and "After" diagnostic models

weaker the result. Setting time is affected also by the length and speed of mixing. The longer and more rapid the mix, the shorter the setting time. Setting time can be accelerated or retarded by using chemical additives. Sodium tetraborate (Borax) will retard setting time, whereas salts, such as sodium chloride or potassium sulfate, in small quantities, will accelerate the set.

Accurate models demand that gypsum products, when set, not change their shape. Consequently, the dimensional stability of these products is important. Improper manipulation can cause changes in dimension that can result in an inaccurate model from an accurate impression.

Plasters and stone are mixed in a flexible rubber bowl with a stiff spatula. A premeasured amount of water is added to the gypsum product. One difficulty encountered with mixing is the incorporation of air bubbles. These bubbles, however, can be removed by using an automatic vibrator and vibrating the mix until no more bubbles come to the surface. The mix can then be poured or shaped as needed.

To fill an impression with mixed plaster or stone, hold the tray by the handle and lean the side of the tray against the vibrator. With a mixing spatula, place a small amount of stone or plaster in the most posterior corner of the impression and vibrate the material slowly through the impression. Be careful to fill each tooth area completely to avoid trapping any air. Continue adding small increments until the impression has been filled to its borders. When filled, set impression aside to harden.

When completely set and hardened, gypsum materials may be trimmed with a laboratory model trimmer (Table 7–2). Cast study

TABLE 7–2. STEPS FOR TRIMMING AND FINISHING
DIAGNOSTIC STUDY CASTS

1. Soak models in water for 5 minutes.
2. Remove any excess material that will interfere with proper occlusion then place wax-bite registration and articulate casts.
3. Apply safety glasses and turn on power and water on model trimmer unit.
4. Trim base of mandibular cast parallel to occlusal plane.
5. Art portion is ⅓ of total height and anatomical portion is ⅔ of total height.
6. Trim heel of mandibular cast, then sides of mandibular cast.
7. Trim front of mandibular cast by rounding anterior cut from cuspid to cuspid.
8. Trim heel of maxillary cast, articulate maxillary and mandibular casts together and note corresponding relation between the heels of the maxillary and mandibular casts.
9. Trim sides of maxillary casts at an angle to heel.
10. Trim front of maxillary anteriors to a sharp point. Point should correspond with mid-line and extend distally to center of maxillary cuspids.
11. Trim with lab knife to depths of fold and to produce an over-all smooth esthetic appearance. Fill in voids with soft plaster.
12. Allow study casts to dry thoroughly, polish by rubbing with a soft chamois and label with patients name, age, and date.

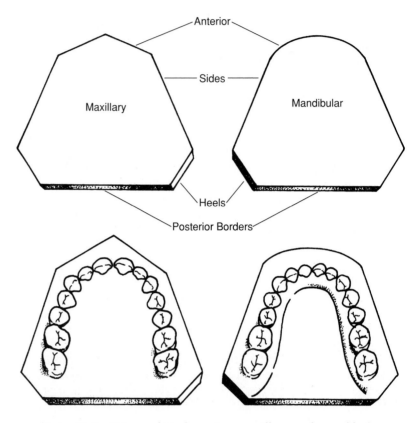

Figure 7–1. Trimmed study casts—maxillary and mandibular.

models are trimmed geometrically and may be polished for esthetics before the patient case presentation appointment (Fig. 7–1).

Special precautions must be taken by the dental auxiliary when working with gypsum products, including the use of protective eyewear during the trimming procedures and while handling the dry powder gypsum plaster or stones. A mask is recommended to prevent inhalation of the fine gypsum powders during manipulation. Auxiliaries should work in well-ventilated laboratory areas equipped with exhaust systems to minimize prolonged exposure to the gypsum materials.

## Summary

- All dental materials are made up of atomic matter.
- Matter exists in three different states: solid, liquid, and gas.
- If heat is given off, the reaction is exothermic.
- If heat is absorbed, the reaction is endothermic.
- The main constituent of all plasters and stones is calcium sulfate hemihydrate.
- Use of a mask is recommended to prevent inhalation of fine gypsum powders during manipulation.
- Class I stone is used mainly for pouring casts.
- Class II stone (high-strength stone) is used to make dies.
- Water/powder ratios are important and affect gypsum product setting times.
- To remove entrapped air bubbles from mix, place mixing bowl on automatic vibrator and vibrate mix well.

■ Add small increments of mixed stone or plaster into an impression to avoid trapping any air.
■ Models may be trimmed geometrically on a model trimmer. Protective eyewear is required when using a model trimmer.

## IV. RESTORATIVE MATERIALS

Direct restorative materials are used to replace tooth structure that has been naturally or mechanically removed. The restorative materials are used for permanent restorations.

Dental amalgam, a combination of mercury with a silver-tin alloy containing small amounts of copper and zinc, is the material of choice for approximately 75% of all dental restorations. Each constituent of the material adds properties to the final product. Silver adds strength and decreases flow. Tin tends to reduce expansion, but also reduces strength. Zinc acts as a deoxidizer. Copper improves strength and hardness. High-copper alloys are being manufactured. The high-copper alloys contain a greater percentage of copper per weight.

Mercury wets the alloy particles and chemically reacts with the alloy to begin the hardening process.

Mercury is mixed with the metallic alloy, which is produced in different forms ranging from a fine powder to a compressed pellet or sphere. The process of mixing together silver alloy particles with liquid mercury is called **trituration.** Trituration may occur by using a mechanical amalgamator. Premeasured capsules eliminate direct contact with free mercury and ensure an accurate alloy-mercury ratio. Once the premeasured capsules are activated, they may be placed in the amalgamator for trituration to occur. The resulting amalgam is plastic and can be inserted, condensed, and carved easily in the cavity preparation.

Undertrituration or overtrituration diminishes the properties of amalgam. Undertriturated amalgam becomes crumbly, is difficult to manipulate, and is diminished in strength. Overtriturated amalgam is runny in consistency and is difficult to manipulate. Amalgam is widely used for its high compressive strength, relative inexpensiveness, and ease of manipulation.

**Mercury toxicity** awareness can reduce potential related occupational hazards from mercury contamination in the dental office. Mercury contamination may occur from accidental spills and direct contact with the liquid metal. Heating of contaminated amalgam carrier instruments and inhaling the mercury vapors are other methods of mercury toxicity. Mulling the amalgam in bare hands, improper disposal methods of unwanted mercury scraps, mechanical amalgamator leakage, and working in a nonventilated area with metal exposure also are occupational hazards.

Symptoms of mercury toxicity range from chronic headaches and fatigue to more serious health problems related to kidney dysfunctions, tremors, speech disorders, and death. Special precautions must be taken by the dental auxiliary when handling mercury to avoid potential health risks.

Mercury Toxicity Preventive Measures:

1. Avoid handling fresh alloy and direct contact with mercury.
2. Properly dispose of scrap mercury, preferably in a closed container with a liquid solution.

---

### Metal Components of Amalgam

Silver—adds strength and decreases flow
Tin—reduces expansion and strength
Zinc—acts as a deoxidizer
Copper—improves strength and hardness
Mercury—wets alloy, begins hardening process

---

### Symptoms of Mercury Toxicity

Chronic headaches
Fatigue
Kidney dysfunction
Tremors
Speech disorders

3. Work in a well-ventilated area of the office when handling mercury materials. Use gloves.
4. Pick up spilled mercury immediately with special office emergency spill kits.
5. Use tightly sealed capsules during amalgamation.
6. When removing old amalgam restorations, use the high-speed evacuator and a water spray. Masks and face shields should be worn.

# V.   COMPOSITE RESIN MATERIALS

▶ **Composite** resins are used primarily for anterior restorations. In addition, composite resins can be used to correct anomalies of enamel development and other esthetic problems and to bond orthodontic brackets. Composites contain a monomer or an aromatic dimethacrylate (most commonly BIS-GMA), an accelerator, organic peroxide, and a filler, such as quartz or glass. Catalysts that quicken setting time vary according to the system used. These systems include self-curing, ultraviolet light curing, and visible light curing. Composite is moderately strong and can be easily manipulated. However, it can be abraded and lose its finish easily.

If the composite is a paste/paste self-curing system, it is mixed by placing equal portions of catalyst and base on a small mixing pad. Different sides of double-ended plastic spatulas are used to avoid contaminating the materials. The two pastes are incorporated into a homogeneous mixture. Etching the enamel walls of the preparation with phosphoric acid before insertion of the composite improves retention and diminishes marginal leakage. Placement of the mixed composite resin material is done with a plastic placement instrument. A celluloid matrix strip is used if indicated for Class III restorations. Composite resin restorative materials should not be manipulated with metal instruments.

# VI.   PIT AND FISSURE SEALANTS

Pit and fissure sealants are synthetic resins that play an important role in preventive dental procedures. The resin is an organic polymer that bonds to the enamel surface by penetrating into the enamel ▶ pores created on the tooth as a result of **acid etching** techniques with phosphoric acid. The resin material is an unfilled BIS-GMA ▶ resin that reacts with a **light-cured polymerization** system or the peroxide-amine technique of polymerization. Pit and fissure resins exhibit properties of low viscosity, which allow the material to flow easily over the tooth. Sealants are subject to occlusal wear and must be examined at regular recall intervals.

# VII.   BONDING AGENTS

## A.   ENAMEL BONDING AGENTS

Enamel bonding agents are used to repair ortho brackets and fractured anterior teeth and for esthetics. The synthetic type of bonding resin exhibits similar chemical and physical properties to the composite resins and the pit and fissure sealants. Before placement of a bonding agent, it is necessary to acid etch the tooth surface.

## B. DENTIN BONDING AGENTS

Dentin bonding agents are used to seal the dentinal tubules of a prepared tooth to prevent postoperative sensitivity to the pulp. Dentin bonding systems may be either light-cured or self-cured. Specialized dentin bonding systems may also improve retention of cast metal restorations and amalgams to prevent micro-leakage or recurrent decay. Acid etching is required prior to placement of a dentin bonding agent. Acid etching dissolves the enamel prisms and creates a roughened surface with microscopic enamel surface tags which allow the bonding materials to adhere (penetrate) the tooth surface.

## VIII. ACRYLIC RESINS

Acrylic resins are polymeric restorative materials used in anterior teeth. The resins come in a powder and liquid form. The liquid is a **monomer** comprised of methyl methylacrylate (hydroquinone), an ◀ accelerator, and an organic sulfonic acid. The powder is a **polymer** ◀ of polymethyl methacrylate, benzoyl peroxide (a catalyst), and metal oxides. The material has the ability to withstand fracture and is available in a wide range of shades. Disadvantages include low resistance to wear and an inability to prevent recurring caries. In addition, the restoration can change shape over time and alternately expand and contract. This results in an exchange of fluids in the margins, a process known as percolation. Temporary crowns are fabricated from acrylic resin, and permanent crowns are often faced with acrylic veneers.

There are two techniques of applying direct acrylic resins to a tooth preparation: brush, or Nealon, and bulk techniques. In the brush technique, liquid and powder are placed into separate dappen dishes. A sable brush is dipped into the liquid and then into the powder, and the acrylic bead is placed into the tooth preparation. This method is repeated until the tooth is fully restored.

In the bulk technique, powder and liquid are mixed in a single dappen dish until a doughlike consistency is obtained. The mix is placed in the tooth preparation with a plastic instrument and is held in place with a matrix until it is set.

## Summary

- Restorative materials are used for permanent restorations.
- Trituration is the process of mixing together silver alloy particles with liquid mercury.
- Amalgam is widely used for its high compressive strength.
- Mercury contamination may occur from accidental spills and direct contact with the liquid metal.
- Improper disposal methods of unwanted mercury scraps pose an occupational hazard.
- Composite resins are used primarily for anterior restorations.
- Composites exhibit light-cured or self-curing properties.

- Etching with phosphoric acid is required before insertion of a composite.
- Celluloid matrix strips are used for proximal composite restorations.
- Composites should not be mixed with metallic instruments.
- Pit and fissure sealants are subject to occlusal wear and must be examined at regular recall intervals.
- Before a bonding agent is placed, it is necessary to acid etch the tooth surface.
- Dentin bonding agents are used to seal the dentinal tubules of a prepared tooth to prevent postoperative sensitivity to the pulp.
- Specialized dentin bonding agents may be used to improve the retention of cast metal restorations.
- Acrylic resins are polymeric restorative materials used in anterior teeth. The resins come in a powder/liquid form.

# IX.   DENTAL CEMENTS

Cements in dentistry are used as luting agents for permanent restorations and orthodontic bands, as temporary restorations, and as thermal insulators for the pulp under metallic restorations.

## A.   ZINC PHOSPHATE CEMENT

Zinc phosphate cement is a powder/liquid system. The powder is composed of zinc oxide and magnesium oxide, and the liquid contains phosphoric acid, water, and a small amount of aluminum phosphate. Zinc phosphate cements are high in acidity and can cause pulpal damage if not mixed properly. As is true of all cements, they are soluble in oral fluids and will not adhere to tooth structure under moist conditions.

Advantages of zinc phosphate cement are its properties of malleability and high compressive strength. Setting time can be controlled, allowing the dentist flexibility to use the material for various procedures simultaneously, such as cementation of several orthodontic bands from one single mix.

Zinc phosphate cement is mixed on a dry, cool glass slab with a metal spatula. Drops of the liquid are placed on the glass slab, and small increments of powder are incorporated, using a rotary motion, with the spatula held flat against the glass slab. The material is mixed over a large area of the glass slab in order to dissipate heat. The correct consistency for cementation can be determined by checking the flow of the mix. A thinner mix is desired for final luting procedures, and a thicker mix is used for insulating bases under restorations.

## B.   GLASS IONOMER CEMENTS

Glass ionomer cements may be used for permanent luting procedures of dental crowns, fixed bridgework, and as a restorative material for conservative Class V restorations. The composition of the glass ionomer cement powder is an aluminosilicate glass structure, and the liquid composition is a polycarboxylate copolymer in an aqueous solution. Glass ionomer cements exhibit high compressive strength, and are more resistant to the effects of erosion in the oral cavity. The glass ionomer cements also have the ability to form a

---

**Dental Cements**

Zinc Phosphate Cement
Glass Ionomer
Zinc Oxide Eugenol
Polycarboxylate

stronger adhesive bond to dentin and enamel, creating a tighter seal and inhibiting secondary decay. Glass ionomer cements are cariostatic due to their ability to release fluoride ions incorporated in the powder composition of the ionomer cements used for permanent restorations of anterior teeth.

Glass ionomer cements can be mixed on a cool glass slab or on a nonabsorbent paper pad. The powder is incorporated into the liquid rapidly while spatulating. Unlike zinc phosphate cements, which incorporate several small increments of powder over a longer spatulation period, the glass ionomers incorporate three to four large increments of powder over a 45-second time period of mixing. Strict adherence to procedures to prevent moisture contamination before final cementation must be followed when working with the glass ionomers. Premature moisture contact may contribute to tooth hypersensitivity and microleakage.

Pre-measured capsules containing the manufacturer's recommended powder/liquid ratio are also available. These capsules require the use of the manufacturer's activator device for releasing the liquid into the powder capsule. The capsule is then placed in a high-speed amalgamator for trituration. A specialized dispenser loading gun is used for final release of the mixed glass ionomer cement.

## C. ZINC OXIDE-EUGENOL

Zinc oxide-eugenol (ZOE) is usually dispensed in a powder/liquid system. The powder is composed of zinc oxide, which can contain a small amount of fillers and zinc salts, and the liquid is eugenol (oil of cloves). This cement has a sedative effect on the pulpal tissues and is used to ameliorate pain from toothaches. ZOE is easy to manipulate, and setting can be controlled by accelerators, decreasing moisture, or altering the powder/liquid ratio. ZOE has low compressive strength and is highly soluble in oral fluids. Consequently, it is not used in final restorations. ZOE may be used as an insulating base under restorations and for cementation of temporary crowns or as a sedative temporary dressing.

ZOE is mixed by adding the powder to the liquid in small amounts and vigorously spatulating the mix with a metal spatula on an oil-impervious paper pad or glass slab until the desired thickness is obtained. As with all cements, the more powder used, the stronger the material.

Improved zinc oxide-eugenol also comes in a strengthened form, which is reinforced with ortho-ethoxybenzoic acid (EBA). It is a powder/liquid system that is easy to manipulate, flows readily under pressure, and has a long working time. It achieves adequate strength only if there is a high powder/liquid ratio. The material is mixed on a glass slab, and powder is added to the liquid. The mix is then spatulated vigorously under pressure for 2 minutes to achieve fluidity. Lowering the temperature of the glass slab will slow the setting of the cement. EBA cements are used for luting of permanent castings such as inlays, crowns, and bridges.

## D. POLYCARBOXYLATE CEMENT

Polycarboxylate cement, also referred to as carboxylate and polyacrylate, is a powder/liquid system used for luting or orthodontic band cementation. The powder consists mainly of zinc oxide, with some magnesium oxide and aluminum oxide. The liquid contains poly-acrylic and organic acids in an aqueous solution. This cement is not irritating to pulpal tissue, has relatively low solubility in oral fluids, and adheres best to clean enamel. One disadvantage is its short working time.

Polycarboxylate cement can be mixed on a paper pad or glass slab. When mixed on a cool glass slab, working time may be increased. The powder is incorporated into the liquid in large increments and spatulated quickly until homogeneous. Failure to mix the cement rapidly will produce a mix with a dull appearance and tacky consistency unsuitable for cementation procedures of permanent castings.

## Summary

- Dental cements may be used for luting, temporary restorations, and as thermal insulators for the pulp.
- Zinc phosphate cement is mixed on a dry, cool glass slab with a metal spatula.
- A thin mix is desired for luting procedures and a thick mix is used for insulating bases under metallic restorations.
- Glass ionomer cements are cariostatic because of their ability to release fluoride ions.
- Glass ionomer cements may be mixed on a nonabsorbent paper pad over a 45-second time period or in a high-speed amalgamator, if in capsule form.
- ZOE has a sedative effect on the pulp and is used to ameliorate pain from toothaches.
- ZOE has low compressive strength and may be used as a sedative temporary dressing or for temporary crown cementation.
- EBA cements are stronger and are used for luting or permanent castings.
- Polycarboxylate cements have a short working time.

## X.   VARNISHES AND LINERS

Varnishes and liners are used to insulate pulpal tissue. Varnish is a coating material, consisting mainly of a natural gum or a synthetic resin in an organic solvent solution. Varnishes block irritating chemicals contained in restorative materials from entering the dentinal tubules and affecting the pulp.

The technique for using varnish involves dipping a cotton pledget into the varnish, removing the excess, and coating the walls of the cavity. Application of the varnish may also be done with a fine brush. At least two coatings of varnish should be applied to cover all walls of the cavity preparation. Setting time is approximately 15 to 30 seconds.

Calcium hydroxide is a liner available in liquid/paste or paste/paste form. The paste hardens and forms a thin layer over the dentin. It stimulates the formation of secondary dentin, which acts as additional protection for the pulp. It also forms a barrier against irritants from marginal leakage of restorative materials. This material must be used on dentin only, since placement on enamel walls of cavity preparations can contribute to marginal leakage of final restorations as a result of its high degree of solubility in oral fluids.

Calcium hydroxide is mixed on a paper pad with a small, ball-shaped metal applicator. Equal amounts of the base and catalyst are extruded onto the mixing pad and rapidly mixed until homogeneous. The cavity liner may be applied with the same instrument used for mixing or with an explorer.

## XI.  DENTAL PORCELAIN

Dental porcelain is an esthetic material widely used in final restorations. It is highly compatible with oral tissues and is resistant to abrasion. It is used in the fabrication of artificial teeth in dentures and crowns, and as a veneer fused to metal copings. Porcelains are classified by the temperature at which they mature. All are made of particles of feldspar and quartz. The feldspar serves as a matrix for the quartz, and the quartz is a strengthener and filler.

Porcelain is highly resistant to the forces of compression but is also highly susceptible to bending forces. Consequently, restorations and tooth preparations must be designed to deemphasize exposure to unnecessary bending forces in the oral cavity.

Porcelain is produced as a powder that is mixed with water to form a pastelike substance that can be molded or condensed into the desired shape. The substance is then fired in a furnace and is subsequently glazed to polish the surface and improve the strength of the restoration. It is important to use minimum amounts of water to avoid shrinkage during the condensation or firing processes.

The finished restoration can then be placed into the mouth. Restorations entirely fabricated from porcelain are used primarily in the anterior portion of the mouth. When used for posterior restorations, the material is fused to a cast alloy coping that fits the prepared tooth or teeth.

## XII.  BLEACHING AGENTS

A variety of bleaching methods exist to improve the appearance (color) of anterior teeth. Bleaching methods include in-office bleaching methods directed under the supervision of the dentist and home bleaching kits that may be used by the patient without direct supervision.

Bleaching agents include gels or solutions which are applied in a series of appointments on pre-fabricated custom plastic trays. Bleaching agents include a high percentage of hydrogen peroxide and may require the use of a curing light.

Bleaching of an individual tooth which has internal pulpal injury and is diagnosed as non-vital may require in-office bleaching. To remove the darkened discoloration of the tooth, a paste-like substance of sodium perborate and hydrogen peroxide is placed in the tooth pulp chamber and sealed. Patients are reappointed within a week to change the paste-like dressing and the bleaching procedure is repeated until the tooth is no longer discolored.

### Summary

- Varnishes and liners are used to insulate pulpal tissue.
- Varnishes may be applied with a fine brush.
- Calcium hydroxide is a liner which stimulates the formation of secondary dentin.

- Dental porcelain is used in the fabrication of artificial teeth and crowns which are primarily used in the anterior portion of the mouth.
- Bleaching agents include a high percentage of hydrogen peroxide and may require the use of a curing light.
- In-office bleaching of a non-vital tooth may require several visits.

# XIII.   ELASTOMERIC IMPRESSION MATERIALS

| Elastomers |
|---|
| Polysulfide |
| Silicone |
| Polyvinylsiloxane |
| Polyether |

Impression materials are used in dentistry to obtain accurate, detailed negative images of hard and soft oral tissues. **Elastomers** are elastic impression materials manufactured from synthetic rubber and appear soft and rubberlike when set. Elastomeric impression materials possess low distortion properties once an impression has been taken and the material sets.

Elastomeric impression materials are self-curing and are available as a base/catalyst system. The base portion of the elastomeric material is either putty-like or paste-like. The catalyst (accelerator) is available as either a liquid or paste. Elastomeric materials cure (polymerize) from a paste into a rubber-like impression material. The material is generally supplied in three forms, light, medium, or heavy body.

## A.   POLYSULFIDE IMPRESSION MATERIAL

Polysulfide impression material, also known as mercaptan (rubber base), produces an impression through the chemical process of polymerization, which is the chemical reaction whereby single units (monomers) link to form larger units (polymers).

The material is supplied in two tubes of paste. One tube, the base, contains the basic reactive substance, a low molecular weight polysulfide polymer, and fillers. The other tube, the accelerator, contains lead peroxide and sulfur, which actually cause the vulcanization reaction that forms a longer-chain rubber material.

The material is mixed by spatulating equal lengths of base and accelerator on a paper pad for 45 to 60 seconds. The material, homogenized in color, is then placed in a preformed custom or stock tray and inserted into the patient's mouth. The material sets in about 6 to 8 minutes and is very accurate. It is used to take final impressions for models on which crowns, bridges, inlays, and partial dentures are fabricated. The material's disadvantages are its offensive smell, staining ability, and inconsistent setting time, which is shortened by increased temperature and humidity.

## B.   SILICONE IMPRESSION MATERIAL

Silicone impression material is similar to polysulfide material in many ways. It sets via a polymerization reaction in 6 to 8 minutes and is supplied in two tubes (a base and a catalyst). It is carried to the mouth in the same type of tray as polysulfide and is used for the same purposes. The base, a paste, contains a polymer, dimethylsilocaine, and an organic filler. The catalyst, usually a liquid, contains tin octoate that initiates the reaction. The base is dispensed onto a paper pad, and the catalyst is added. The material is spatulated for about a minute until a homogeneous color results. Its color and odor are among its advantages, and its disadvantages include a shorter shelf-life than that of other impression materials. Silicone is also available in a putty/wash system. The putty is mixed with a liquid catalyst. The putty contains up to 70% fillers as compared with the 45% of the regular-bodied silicone. After the putty has set, a wash material (a fluid silicone base mixed with the same liquid catalyst) is smoothed over the putty impression and placed over the teeth. This process results in an accurate, detailed impression.

## C.   POLYVINYLSILOXANE IMPRESSION MATERIAL

Polyvinylsiloxane, or polysiloxane, is also known as an addition re-action silicone impression material. The impression material is available as a two-paste system which is mixed using a specialized dispenser gun that allows twin tubes of catalyst and base to be automatically mixed in the dispensing tip of the "extruder dual cartridge impression gun."

Contact with latex gloves may retard the setting time of the polyvinylsiloxane heavy bodied putty tray material. When handling the putty impression, material vinyl overgloves are recommended.

## D.   POLYETHER IMPRESSION MATERIAL

Polyether impression materials are the third impression material in the elastomeric group and are similar to polysulfide and silicone in their polymerization reaction. However, when polyether is used, the impression can be recorded in a single step without a second wash impression. The material is supplied in two tubes. The base contains a polyether polymer, and the accelerator is a sulfonic acid ester. The materials are dispensed in equal lengths onto a paper mixing pad and spatulated for about 45 to 60 seconds until a homogeneous color is attained. Setting time is 2-1/2 to 3 minutes. Polyether materials are highly accurate and are used for the same purposes as other elastic impression materials. A factor to be considered when using these materials is the difficulty of removing set impressions from the patient's mouth because polyether impression materials exhibit a high degree of stiffness. A body modifier, or thinner, may be incorporated to reduce the stiffness. The polyether chemistry of this material may cause hypersensitivity in certain individuals.

### Summary

- Elastomeric impression materials are self-curing and are available as a base/catalyst system.
- Elastomeric materials polymerize from a paste into a rubber-like impression material.
- Polysulfide impression materials are also known as mercaptan (rubber base).
- Polysulfide impression materials are used to take final impressions for crowns, bridges, and inlays.
- Silicone impression materials polymerize in 6 to 8 minutes.
- Vinyl gloves are recommended when working with polyvinyl-siloxane impression materials.
- Polyether impression materials exhibit a high degree of stiffness.

# XIV.   ELASTIC IMPRESSION MATERIALS

## A.   REVERSIBLE HYDROCOLLOID

Reversible, or agar, hydrocolloid is a thermoelastic material in which an impression is recorded through the physical change of agar from a sol to a gel. Agar hydrocolloid is packaged in tubes and is composed of 80% to 85% water, 12% to 15% agar, a small percentage of sodium tetraborate (Borax), which adds strength, and 2% potassium sulfate, which enhances proper setting. Hydrocolloid is prepared by boiling in a waterbath conditioner at 212°F. The hydrocolloid may then be stored at 150°F in the conditioning unit storage bath. Before the impression is taken, it is placed in water-cooled trays and immersed in the conditioning unit tempering bath to bring the material to a tolerable temperature for contact with the oral tissues.

Agar hydrocolloids are extremely accurate materials and are used for final impressions to make models for the fabrication of partial dentures, crowns, bridges, and inlays. The material has a low tear strength and the potential for high-dimensional change resulting from imbibition (the taking up of water). To minimize dimensional distortions, the impression should be poured immediately.

## B.   IRREVERSIBLE HYDROCOLLOID-ALGINATE

▶ Irreversible, or **alginate,** hydrocolloid is a material that produces an impression through the process of chemical change. Mixing the soluble sodium alginate, which also contains calcium sulfate, with water results in the formation of an insoluble calcium alginate gel. Trisodium phosphate in the powder acts as a retardant and permits more working time. The remaining ingredients include diatomaceous earth, which acts as a filler; a complex fluoride compound, which helps create adequate surface strength for the gypsum model materials; a coloring agent; and flavor additives.

The material is manipulated by first placing the powder, measured in scoops, into a rubber mixing bowl. A measured amount of water at room temperature (70°F) is then added, and the mix is spatulated in a whipping motion until a homogeneous sol is formed. The temperature of the water is extremely important, since higher temperatures shorten working and setting times. The mix is placed immediately in a fitted perforated or rim-locked tray.

Alginate is not as accurate in recording fine detail as other impression materials (eg, reversible hydrocolloids), and as a result, it is used to take impressions for study models used in diagnosis and the fabrication of orthodontic appliances and night guards. The material can be used to take final impressions for partial dentures. In addition to being inexpensive, alginate is easy to manipulate. It has a low tear ▶ strength and is not dimensionally stable because of **syneresis** (loss of water).

If an alginate impression is stored in a very wet paper towel, ▶ distortion and expansion may occur due to **imbibition.** It is best to store the impression in a sealed container or sealed plastic bag with a damp paper towel or damp 4×4 gauze square, which creates an atmosphere of 100% relative humidity. Appropriate disinfection measures must be performed if sending alginate impressions to be poured at a commercial dental laboratory. Read manufacturer's instructions for recommendations regarding an approved surface disinfectant which may be sprayed on the alginate impression material safely without causing distortion or damage to the impression.

## Summary

- Agar hydrocolloids are extremely accurate materials and are used for final impressions.
- Reversible agar hydrocolloids undergo a physical change from sol to gel.
- Water-cooled trays are required for hydrocolloids.
- Hydrocolloid impression materials should be poured immediately. Imbibition can cause dimensional distortion.
- Irreversible hydrocolloid (alginate) contains diatomaceous earth, which acts as a filler.
- Perforated or rim-locked trays are used for alginate impressions.
- Alginate is mixed in a rubber mixing bowl with a measured amount of room temperature water. A metal spatula is used to whip the material into a homogenous sol.
- Alginate has a low tear strength and will undergo syneresis if not stored properly prior to pouring.
- Disinfection measures must be performed when sending alginate impressions to a commercial dental laboratory.

## XV.   PLASTIC IMPRESSION MATERIALS

### A.   DENTAL COMPOUND

Thermal modeling plastic, or dental compound, is a material that produces an impression through a physical change of shape at a specific temperature. It is comprised of various thermoplastic resins, waxes, fillers, and coloring agents. Thermal modeling plastics are used to take preliminary impressions for full or partial dentures and for final impressions of single crown preparations. When denture impressions are desired, compound shaped wafers or cakes are used. When single crown impressions are desired, compound sticks are used. Dental compound has low thermal conductivity and should be heated slowly and evenly.

When the material is prepared for a preliminary impression, it should be softened in a waterbath at 130°F until it can be kneaded. The compound should not remain in the water for too long a period since some of the necessary ingredients may dissolve and a grainy material may result. Similarly, when stick compound is warmed over a flame, it should be heated in a manner that prevents melting or dripping in order to maintain suitable flow properties. The materials are impressed against the mouth tissues while still warm and flowing (113°F). By the time the material reaches mouth temperature (98.6°F), it exhibits very little flow. Corrective washes (or final impressions) are taken over denture impressions.

### B.   DENTAL WAXES

Dental waxes are thermoplastic materials that come in many forms and are used for various procedures. They are categorized into three groups: pattern waxes, processing waxes, and impression waxes. These dental waxes are composed of a combination of materials that form organic polymers. Ingredients include resins, oils, fat, gums, pigments, and natural and synthetic waxes.

1. **Pattern waxes** are used to form the patterns from which metal or resin restorations are cast. Examples of pattern waxes are inlay wax, used to produce patterns for inlays, crowns, and pontics, and casting wax, used to create the pattern for the metal framework of a removable prosthesis.
2. **Processing waxes** are waxes used in the laboratory. Examples include boxing wax, used to prepare gypsum models, sticky wax, used to reattach plaster impressions, and periphery wax, used to adjust trays to the appropriate size.
3. **Impression wax** manufactured in various arch shapes is used when taking full denture impressions. Examples include corrective impression wax, used to record or fill specific areas of impressions made from other materials when minute detail is desired, and bite registration wax and wafer impression wax, used to record occlusal registration.

## C.   ZINC OXIDE-EUGENOL IMPRESSION PASTES

Zinc oxide-eugenol (ZOE) impression pastes are used for secondary impressions. ZOE functions as a final wash and is inserted into a preliminary impression tray. It is used most often for full denture impressions in a preformed tray. The material is dispensed in a paste/paste system and mixed on oil-impervious paper. Initial setting time is approximately 3 to 6 minutes, and final set ranges from 10 to 15 minutes. Setting time can be accelerated using a zinc acetate salt or a drop of water. Although the material is dimensionally stable, ZOE impression paste can irritate oral tissues because of its eugenol constituent, which can cause burning or stinging.

## XVI.   ACRYLIC DENTURE BASE RESINS

Denture bases are made from acrylic resins because of the material's dimensional stability, esthetic appearance, ability to absorb shock, and weight. Self-curing acrylic resins can be worked and set at room temperature and are often used to repair dentures that have broken. Acrylic resins are also used to rebase and reline dentures. Because the oral tissues on which the dentures rest change with time, dentures must sometimes be adapted to accommodate these changes. When dentures are rebased, the old base is used as an impression tray. The former base is replaced with one made from a new impression. The same teeth are used for the new base.

When minor changes occur in the oral tissues, a denture can be relined rather than rebased. The existing base is used to take an impression, and the appropriate amount of acrylic is added to accommodate the changes.

# XVII.   CUSTOM TRAYS

Self-cured acrylic resins are used to make custom trays for impressions. These trays produce high-quality impressions because they are accurate replications of individual oral tissues.

An electric vacuum former can also be used to heat a sheet of plastic material to fabricate custom made bleaching trays, or night guards and mouth guards.

Light-cured resins, or thermoplastic materials, are also used to fabricate custom trays.

The following criteria is necessary for the accurate construction of a custom tray:

1. Eliminate all signs of undercuts in the dental cast prior to preparation.
2. Place an appropriate spacer and spacer stops to prevent tray from seating incorrectly. Custom tray should be able to cover the patient's dental arch adequately.
3. If required, fabricate a handle in the anterior part of the tray.
4. Use a separating medium during fabrication to facilitate tray removal from the cast.
5. Smooth rough tray edges with lab knife and polish.
6. Clean tissue side of tray and disinfect before seating in the patient's mouth.
7. Custom tray should provide strength, durability, and comfort during use.

## Summary

- Dental compound is used to take preliminary impressions for full or partial dentures.
- Casting wax is used to form the patterns for the metal framework or a removable prosthesis.
- Inlay wax is used to produce patterns for inlays, crowns, and pontics.
- Boxing wax is used to prepare gypsum models.
- Periphery wax is used to adjust impression trays.
- A bite registration is taken using an arch shaped wax.
- ZOE impression pastes are used for full denture impressions in a preformed tray.
- Self-curing acrylic resins are used to repair dentures that have broken.
- Dentures can be relined if there are minor changes in the oral tissues.
- An electric vacuum former can be used to heat a sheet of plastic material to fabricate custom made bleaching trays, night guards, and mouth protectors.

# XVIII.   CAST GOLD RESTORATIONS

Often, in a severely deteriorated tooth that is missing a considerable amount of structure, direct filling materials, such as amalgam, cannot be used because they would be unable to withstand masticatory forces. Rather, stronger cast restorations are fabricated.

TABLE 7–3.  CLASSIFICATION OF CASTING GOLD ALLOYS

Type I alloys are soft and are used for simple inlays
Type II alloys are harder, can be used for two and three surface inlays, and
  are the most common alloys used for operative procedures
Type III alloys are used for fixed prostheses, and crown and bridge abutments
Type IV alloys are extra hard and are used for denture frameworks

The use of pure metal in dentistry is quite limited. The most commonly used materials are combinations of two or more metals, known as alloys. Casting gold alloys may contain gold, silver, copper, palladium, platinum, and zinc. Gold resists tarnish and corrosion and contributes ductility and malleability to the alloy. Silver reduces the deep yellow color of gold and red tint of copper by its natural gray color. Copper increases the strength and hardness of the alloy and generally reduces the melting point. Platinum increases the strength, hardness, and resistance to tarnish and corrosion. Like silver, it also helps whiten the color. Palladium increases the melting point, hardens the compound, and whitens the alloy. Zinc acts as a scavenger and reacts with any oxides first, and increases the casting ability of the alloy. It also reduces the melting point.

Gold alloys are cast into inlays, crowns, bridges, and partial denture frameworks. The base metal alloys, such as cobalt chromium, are used in constructing partial denture frameworks.

Gold alloy materials are classified according to gold content and hardness, which correlates to material strength. There are four types of dental gold alloys (Table 7–3).

## XIX.  ABRASIVE MATERIALS

The polishing process may take place either intraorally or in a laboratory. If the polishing is done in the mouth, caution must be taken to prevent overheating the tooth and consequently damaging vital tissues. Common abrasive materials used in dentistry include diamond stones, wheels, and discs, carborundum wheels and discs, aluminum oxide discs, and quartz sandpaper discs. Most of these agents are available in graduated degrees of abrasiveness.

Abrasives and polishing agents can be mixed with a lubricant such as water or glycerin to produce a slurry or paste. Dentures are usually finished by buffing with an abrasive slurry on a laboratory type lathe buffing wheel. During a dental prophylaxis, teeth are polished with a rubber cup using a slurry-like abrasive paste.

Additional types of intraoral abrasives include tin oxide, used for polishing metallic restorations, and flour of pumice-fine grit, used for polishing extrinsic stains from the teeth.

Laboratory abrasives include rouge, used for polishing gold and other precious metal alloys, and laboratory coarse grade pumice, used for final finishing and polishing procedures.

### Summary

■ Casting gold alloys contain gold, silver, copper, palladium, platinum, and zinc.
■ Gold resists tarnish and corrosion.

- Gold alloys are cast into inlays, crowns, bridges, and partial denture frameworks.
- There are 4 types of gold alloys.
- Caution must be taken if using abrasives in the mouth to prevent overheating the teeth.
- Abrasives and polishing agents can be mixed with a lubricant such as water.
- Dentures are finished by buffing with an abrasive slurry on a laboratory lathe buffing wheel.
- Tin oxide is used for polishing metallic restorations.
- Flour of pumice is used for polishing extrinsic stains from teeth.

# XX. ENDODONTIC SEDATIVE & PALLIATIVE MATERIALS

## A. ENDODONTIC MATERIALS

Endodontic materials are used to treat the dental pulp and canals of teeth. Sodium hypochlorite is an antibacterial irrigating solution that is used to flush the canals of teeth which have received endodontic treatment.

After the canals have been thoroughly debrided, shaped, and dried by the dentist, the assistant may prepare the endodontic sealer. Obturation, or filling of the canal, is done with gutta percha. The endodontic sealer is mixed on a sterile glass slab prior to final placement of the gutta percha point to create a seal at the apical foramen of the root canal. The sealer is applied with an endodontic file prior to placement of the gutta percha point. The gutta percha point is then condensed into the canal with endodontic spreaders or pluggers. The tooth is sealed with a temporary cement and the patient is rescheduled for post-operative evaluation and final coverage with a permanent restoration.

## B. POST-EXTRACTION DRESSINGS

Post-extraction dressings are used as a palliative treatment to alleviate the discomfort of a dry socket (alveolitis) after an extraction. Dental materials include a warm saline solution for irrigating and cleaning the socket area. A disposable irrigating type of syringe is used for this procedure. Iodoform gauze and a medicated dressing which may contain benzocaine are also applied to the affected area and packed gently into the open socket. The patient should be rescheduled and the procedure repeated as needed until discomfort is diminished.

## C. PERIODONTAL SURGICAL DRESSINGS

Periodontal dressings are used after periodontal surgery to protect the surgical site from trauma and minimize post-operative discomfort. Periodontal dressing materials come as a non-eugenol two paste system (base and accelerator) which is mixed on a paper mixing pad into a putty-like consistency and then applied over the surgical site. Light cured single-dose syringe-type dispenser perio dressings are also available.

A powder/liquid zinc oxide eugenol dressing material is also available and may be mixed ahead of time into a putty-like roll and wrapped in wax paper for storage in the refrigerator for future use. The eugenol constituents in this material may cause tissue irritation to the surgical site.

## Summary

- Endodontic materials are used to treat the dental pulp and canals of teeth.
- Obturation, or filling of a root canal, is done with gutta percha and an endodontic sealer.
- Post-extraction dressings are used as a palliative treatment to alleviate the discomfort of a dry socket (alveolitis).
- Iodoform gauze and a medicated dressing containing benzocaine are applied to the dry socket.
- Periodontal dressings are used after periodontal surgery to protect the surgical site from trauma and minimize post-operative discomfort.
- Periodontal dressing materials come as a non-eugenol two paste system or a powder/liquid system.

# Review Questions

1. Discuss how knowledge of the properties of matter relates to dental materials.

2. Describe what is meant by the chemical reaction known as "heat of reaction."

3. Explain why gypsum products must undergo the process of calcination.

4. Identify the classifications of dental stone.

5. Explain how dental plaster or stone is mixed. Discuss the importance of water-to-powder ratios.

6. How do you fill an impression with mixed plaster or stone?

7. Explain how to trim maxillary and mandibular cast study models.

8. List several precautions the dental auxiliary must take when working with gypsum products.

9. What are the metal components of dental amalgam?

10. Distinguish between trituration, overtrituration, and undertrituration.

11. List several preventive measures which can be taken to reduce mercury toxicity.

12. Describe the composition of a composite resin.

13. Why is it necessary to etch the enamel walls of the preparation prior to placement of a composite resin?

14. Discuss the importance of regular recalls as they relate to pit and fissure sealants.

15. What are enamel bonding agents used for?

16. Describe how dentin bonding agents seal dentinal tubules.

17. Discuss the two techniques of applying direct acrylic resins to a tooth preparation.

18. Explain how zinc phosphate cement is mixed.

19. Why are glass ionomer cements cariostatic?

20. Differentiate between ZOE and improved (EBA) zinc oxide-eugenol.

21. What is polycarboxylate cement used for?

22. How do you apply a cavity varnish?

23. Why is calcium hydroxide only applied to the dentinal layer of a prepared tooth?

24. Why is dental porcelain used primarily in the anterior part of the mouth?

25. Discuss the various methods of bleaching teeth. Your answer should include in-office as well as home bleaching kits.

26. Describe the properties of elastomeric impression materials.

27. How are rubber base (mercaptan) impression materials mixed?

28. Identify the advantages and disadvantages of silicone impression material.

29. Why are latex gloves contraindicated for use with polyvinylsiloxane impression material?

30. Identify the advantages and disadvantages of polyether impression materials.

31. Describe the composition of reversible hydrocolloid.

32. Identify the compartments of a conditioning unit and describe the type of impression trays used for reversible hydrocolloid.

33. What are hydrocolloid impression materials primarily used for?

34. Identify the composition of irreversible hydrocolloid-alginate.

35. What is the alginate impression material primarily used for?

36. What is meant by imbibition and syneresis? What is the best way to store an alginate impression?

37. What must you do to an alginate impression before sending it to a commercial dental laboratory?

38. What are thermal modeling plastics used for?

39. Discuss the various types of dental waxes.

40. What is ZOE impression paste used for?

41. Describe the difference between a denture reline and a denture rebase.

42. List the criteria for the accurate construction of a custom tray.

43. What are the four types of dental gold alloys?

44. Differentiate between abrasives used in the laboratory and abrasives used for polishing teeth.

45. What is gutta percha used for?

46. Describe the materials and steps used for treating a dry socket.

47. What types of dental materials are used as a periodontal dressing following periodontal surgery?

# Medical Emergencies

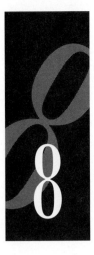

## Key Terms ◀

ALLERGY

ANXIETY

CARDIOPULMONARY RESUSCITA-
TION (CPR)

CONVULSION

CYANOSIS

DIASTOLIC

HYPERVENTILATION

HYPOTENSION

PULSE RATE

SHOCK

SPHYGMOMANOMETER

SYNCOPE

SYSTOLIC

TRENDELENBURG

VASODILATOR

## I. INTRODUCTION

Dental auxiliaries must be properly trained to provide support to the dentist during treatment of an office medical emergency. Medical emergencies may present life-threatening situations, and the auxiliary must be ready to carry out his or her delegated role during an office emergency in a swift and efficient manner. Early recognition of impending medical emergencies and prevention of potential medical complications are the responsibility of each staff member. This chapter provides a synopsis of several specific medical emergencies, including clinical patient signs and symptoms. An overview of related medical emergency procedures and office protocol is given, including medical emergency equipment, supplies, medications, and patient vital signs.

## II.  MEDICAL HISTORY

The best way to treat an emergency is to prevent its occurrence. This can be done by collecting information about patients' medical and dental histories that will inform the office personnel of patients' needs and potential emergency situations. These histories must be updated continuously to provide current information.

Each medical history questionnaire must be reviewed before administering direct patient clinical care. Of special concern to the dental team is patient information about drug allergies, prophylactic antibiotic coverage, history of infectious disease, diseases with related oral manifestations, physiologic changes such as pregnancy, psychologic disorders, and illnesses currently under treatment by the patient's physician that may contraindicate certain dental procedures (Table 8–1). The name and telephone number of the patient's personal physician are vitally important and must be documented clearly on the patient's dental chart.

TABLE 8–1.  MEDICAL HISTORY GUIDELINES

| MEDICAL DISORDER | MEDICAL PREVENTIVE REVIEW |
| --- | --- |
| AIDS | Consult with patient's physician regarding current health status. Patient may be immunocompromised (selective dental treatment). Antibiotic premedication may be required. Transmittable disease. |
| Alcohol/Substance Abuse | Possible liver dysfunction. Increase risk of prolonged clinical duration anesthetics. Increase risk heart valvular damage (antibiotic premedication required). Avoid products containing alcohol. |
| Arthritis/Rheumatism | Possible blood clotting disorder if on long-term medications, antiinflammatory agents, aspirin (salicylates). Corticosteroid therapy long-term requires special precautions. |
| Cancer | Consult with patient's physician regarding current health status. Patient may be on CNS depressants. If immunocompromised selective dental treatment is recommended. Antibiotic premedication may be required due to decreased resistance to infection. |
| Blood Dyscrasias | All bleeding disorders must be evaluated prior to dental treatment. |
| Emphysema | May require supplemental oxygen therapy during dental treatment due to reduced respiratory reserve. Nitrous-oxide is contraindicated. |
| Heart Valve Prosthesis | Recommendation for antibiotic premedication prior to dental treatment. Parenteral prophylactic antibiotic required for extensive surgical dental procedures. |
| Hepatitis | Liver dysfunction. Cautious use of dental anesthetics to avoid overdosage. Clinical duration of anesthetic action is prolonged. Consult with physician. |
| Kidney Problems | May require antibiotic premedication in chronic cases. Consult with physician prior to dental treatment. |
| Rheumatic Fever/Congenital Heart Disease | Consult with patient regarding history rheumatic fever and affects of rheumatic heart disease. Antibiotic premedication required to minimize risk of sub-acute endocarditis (SBE). |
| Tuberculosis | Consult regarding disease status-active/arrested. Transmittable disease. Avoid use of aerosols, cavitron, air-jet polishers. If active disease status use disposable inhalation sedation equipment. |
| Ulcer | Note anxiety levels of patient. Patient may be unable to tolerate additional stress from dental treatment. Medications prescribed include tranquilizers and antacids. |
| Venereal Disease | Observe extraoral and introral tissues for oral lesions. If open weeping lesions defer dental treatment and reschedule patient. |

## III.  VITAL SIGNS

In addition to reviewing the patient's medical history, critical, life-saving information may be obtained by taking and recording the patient's vital signs. Vital signs include blood pressure, pulse rate, respiration rate, and body temperature. This information is often gathered by the dental auxiliary and documented in the patient's dental record for reference by the dentist before dental treatment.

### A.  BLOOD PRESSURE

Blood pressure may be defined as the force or pressure exerted on the walls of the blood vessels from the flow of blood during the contraction and relaxation phase of the heart muscle. Blood pressure is measured during systole, the contraction phase of the heart, and measured as the **systolic** or highest pressure value. During the resting, or relaxation, phase, or diastole, the **diastolic** or lowest blood pressure value is measured.

Blood pressure is measured with special equipment that may include a small portable unit known as a mercury manometer or an aneroid **sphygmomanometer.** The sphygmomanometer consists of an inflatable cuff, pressure gauge or dial, and hand-controlled pressure bulb. The stethoscope is used to listen to the sounds produced by the brachial artery as the blood flow is altered by the pressure exerted from the sphygmomanometer cuff. These sounds are called Korotkoff sounds. The first sound heard through the stethoscope is the systolic blood pressure, and the last sound heard is the diastolic pressure (Fig. 8–1).

The actual measurement of blood pressure is expressed as a fraction, with the systolic pressure over the diastolic pressure (eg, 120/80). The measurement of 120 shows the systolic reading, and the measurement of 80 represents the diastolic pressure reading.

Average systolic values for adults may vary depending on age, height, weight, and health-related complications. An average range may fall between 100 and 140 for systolic pressure and between 60 and 89 for diastolic pressure.

Unusually high blood pressure values (hypertension) or unusually low blood blood pressure values **(hypotension)** should alert the auxiliary to possible medical or drug-related problems. Extremely high systolic and diastolic blood pressure values are of concern because of the increased risk of heart attack and stroke.

### Summary

- The best way to treat an emergency is to prevent its occurrence.
- Medical histories must be updated and reviewed before administering direct patient clinical care.
- Patient's dental chart must include name and telephone number of personal physician.
- Vital signs include blood pressure, pulse rate, respiration rate, and body temperature.
- Blood pressure is measured during systole, the contraction phase of the heart, and recorded as the systolic blood pressure measurement.

**Vital Signs**

Blood pressure
  Systolic
  Diastolic
Pulse rate
  60–100 per minute
  Radial artery pulse point
Respiration rate
  16–20 per minute
Body temperature
  98.6°F or 37°C

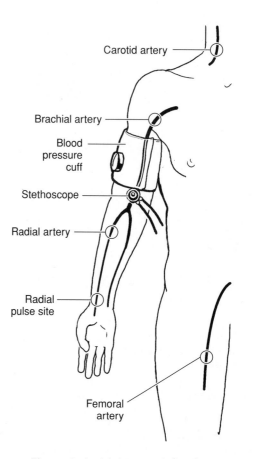

Figure 8–1. Major arterial pulse points.

- During the relaxation phase, diastole, the diastolic blood pressure value is measured.
- Blood pressure is measured with an aneroid sphygmomanometer.
- A stethoscope is used to listen to the Korotkoff sounds produced by the brachial artery as the blood flow is altered by the pressure exerted from the sphygmomanometer cuff.
- Blood pressure is measured as a fraction (eg, 120/80); the 120 indicates the systolic pressure reading and the 80 indicates the diastolic pressure reading.
- High diastolic blood pressure values are known as hypertension.
- Low diastolic blood pressure values are known as hypotension.

## B. PULSE RATE

▶ The average **pulse rate** for adult males is approximately 60 to 100 heartbeats per minute. Women and children generally have slightly higher pulse rates than adult males. Several factors may contribute to slightly higher pulse rates for all patients, including increased activity or exercise, anxiety over impending dental treatment, and certain prescription drugs. The most frequent site for feeling the pulse is at the radial artery, located on the lateral aspect (thumb side) of the wrist (Fig. 8–2). Weak or irregular pulse rates should be recognized

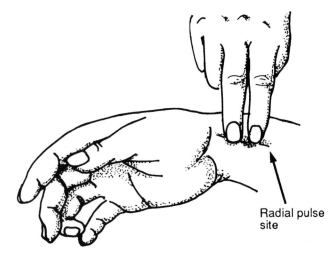

Figure 8–2. Position of fingers to monitor pulse.

and recorded in the patient's dental record. The carotid artery, which is located on the side of the neck, is often used to obtain a pulse rate during cardiopulmonary resuscitation procedures.

## C. RESPIRATION RATE

The average respiration rate for adults is approximately 16 to 20 breaths per minute. Respiration rate may range from 12 to 20 breaths per minute, depending on the patient's age and amount of physical activity or inactivity. Respiration is measured as one complete inspiration and exhalation of air by the lungs. Observations should be made regarding any variations in the rhythm of the respirations or difficult and labored breathing. Unusual sounds, such as wheezing, should be noted.

No movement of the chest or abdomen indicates respiratory failure, and emergency steps to administer **cardiopulmonary resuscitation (CPR)** should begin immediately.

## D. BODY TEMPERATURE

Body temperature is taken orally with a thermometer. The average measurement of body temperature is 98.6°F or 37.0°C. Elevated temperatures may indicate other serious complications or signs of infection and should be treated accordingly. Medical emergencies involving injury to the mouth may require use of the ear thermometer.

### Summary

- Average pulse rate for adult males is 60 to 100 heart beats per minute. Women and children tend to have slightly higher pulse rates.
- The most frequent site for feeling the pulse is at the radial artery, located on the thumb side of the wrist.
- During CPR, the pulse rate is taken at the carotid artery on the side of the neck.
- The average respiration rate for adults is 16–20 breaths per minute.

■ The average measurement of body temperature is 98.6°F. Elevated temperatures may indicate other serious complications.

## IV.   OFFICE PREPARATION FOR AN EMERGENCY

In order to prevent tragic results in an emergency, the office must follow certain procedures. All auxiliaries should be trained to participate in emergency situations and to simulate such situations so that each role is clearly understood.

Emergency support telephone numbers should be prepared in advance and posted in convenient locations near each office telephone. Listings should include local fire departments and emergency room extensions. Telephone numbers of the nearest pharmacy, physician, or medical office, if located in the same building as the dental practice, may be included.

---

**Emergency Support Phone Numbers**

Fire department
Physician
Hospital
Pharmacy
Police department

---

## V.   EMERGENCY KIT AND EQUIPMENT

It is particularly important for all personnel to remain calm and to prevent panic. Procedures should be routine, and materials should be readily available and uncomplicated. An emergency kit should be assembled, and each staff member should be familiar with its use. Basic components of this kit should be emergency equipment, noninjectable drugs, and injectable drugs.

The basic emergency equipment includes an oxygen delivery system, a suction system with tips, syringes, tourniquets, pocket mask, and tube of liquid sugar.

Noninjectable drugs should include oxygen, a respiratory stimulant (aromatic ammonia), a vasodilator (nitroglycerin), a bronchodilator (epinephrine), and an antihypoglycemic (sugar).

Injectable drugs should include epinephrine for severe allergic reactions, diazepam as an anticonvulsant, Benadryl as an antihistamine for mild allergic reactions, hydrocortisone succinate as a corticosteroid, and 50% dextrose glucogen as an antihypoglycemic. These injectable drugs, however, are administered only by specially trained medical or dental personnel.

## VI.   RESPIRATORY EMERGENCIES

In a respiratory emergency, a patient's breathing stops or is reduced to a level at which the body cannot support its oxygen needs. Since nerve tissue can easily be injured from loss of oxygen, an interruption of breathing of 4 to 6 minutes can result in permanent damage. Respiratory failure can occur from obstruction of the airway, hyperventilation, bronchial asthma, heart failure, or acute pulmonary edema.

### A.   HYPERVENTILATION

Dental patients are most likely to experience respiratory difficulties from **hyperventilation** because of **anxiety.** Symptoms include impaired consciousness (loss of consciousness is very rare), lightheadedness, and a feeling of faintness. Breathing may be prolonged,

---

**Respiratory Emergency Treatment**

Hyperventilation—Sit upright and have patient breathe deeply into paper bag to build level of $CO_2$.
Bronchial asthma—Stop treatment, use bronchial dilator.
Heart failure—Sit upright, administer $O_2$, call for emergency medical support.

rapid, or deep. The usual treatment is to discontinue dental treatment, make the patient comfortable, and have the patient breathe into a paper bag to correct respiratory alkalosis by increasing the blood level of $CO_2$.

## B.  BRONCHIAL ASTHMA

Bronchial asthma also may cause respiratory difficulty. These attacks may be precipitated by inhalation of materials that produce an allergic reaction or may be caused by irritating inhalants, infections, or emotional upset. Dental treatment should be stopped, and a bronchial dilator, oxygen, or both may be administered. Symptoms include difficult breathing and wheezing and possible cyanosis, in severe cases.

## C.  HEART FAILURE

Heart failure and acute pulmonary edema also can lead to respiratory problems as a result of the body's inability to transport oxygen adequately. Left-sided heart failure leads to pulmonary congestion, and right-sided failure results in vascular congestion, leading to peripheral edema. Patients suffering from these diseases should not be treated in a supine position. If a problem occurs, seat the patient in an upright position and give oxygen while medical assistance is summoned.

## VII.  ARTIFICIAL RESPIRATION

In cases of respiratory difficulty, when the heart has stopped beating, artificial respiration and CPR should be instituted. CPR requires special training and should be attempted only by trained individuals. Outside emergency medical assistance should be sought as quickly as possible.

The objective of artificial respiration is to maintain an open airway and mechanically breathe for the victim. The following steps should be used in an emergency situation.

> **Cardiopulmonary Resuscitation**
>
> CPR—Requires special training. Objective is to maintain an open airway and mechanically breathe for the victim.

### Steps in Administering Artificial Respiration (If the Patient Has a Pulse)

Mouth-to-mouth and mouth-to-mask

1. Place victim on his or her back on the ground.
2. Kneel perpendicular to the victim's body, next to the head.
3. Wipe any foreign matter from the victim's mouth with two fingers.
4. Open the airway by tipping the victim's head back until the chin is pointing upward (Fig. 8–3).
5. Place your left ear very close to the victim's mouth and look at the chest to check for breathing; feel for pulse.
6. If the victim is not breathing, pinch the nostrils closed with the fingers of the hand on the forehead, and place your mouth over the victim's mouth and deliver two slow full breaths. Do not allow time for the victim's lungs to deflate between breaths.

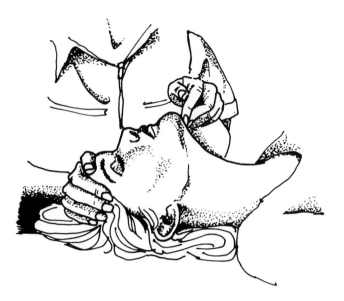

Figure 8–3. Open airway by head tilt and chin tilt.

7. Add a breath every 5 seconds until help has arrived, the victim begins to breathe, or exhaustion overtakes you.
8. Look, listen, and feel for breathing and check the pulse. If the victim begins breathing on his own, discontinue artificial respiration. If the victim is not breathing and has no pulse, begin to administer CPR.

### Steps in Administering Artificial Respiration (If There Is Severe Injury to the Mouth)

Mouth-to-nose

1. Tip the victim's head as for mouth-to-mouth resuscitation.
2. Keep the victim's mouth closed by covering with your hand.
3. Place your mouth over the victim's nose and blow air until the chest rises, one breath every 5 seconds.
4. Place left ear close to the victim's mouth (after removing your hand to allow patient to exhale air) and observe the chest to determine if the patient is breathing. Look, listen, and feel.
5. Add a breath every 5 seconds until help has arrived, the victim begins to breathe, or exhaustion overtakes you.
6. Look, listen, and feel for breathing and check the pulse. If the victim begins breathing on his own, discontinue artificial respiration. If the victim is not breathing and has no pulse, begin to administer CPR.

## VIII. CARDIOVASCULAR EMERGENCY

### A. CONGESTIVE HEART FAILURE (CHF)

Congestive heart failure (CHF) is a broad classification of heart problems that result from an inability of the heart to handle the blood supply. CHF results from several cardiovascular problems. Patients

---

**Cardiovascular Emergency**

CHF—Congestive heart failure
    Sit patient upright and seek emergency medical support.
Myocardial infarction
    Sit patient upright, seek emergency medical support and administer $O_2$.
Angina pectoris
    Sit upright. Administer nitroglycerin sublingually.
Chest pain
    Discontinue treatment and seek emergency medical support.

suffering from this disability usually have trouble lying in a supine position because of fluid retention in the lungs.

Congestive heart failure is usually the outcome of other cardiovascular diseases, most importantly coronary heart disease (CHD), which includes three major categories: arteriosclerotic heart disease (ASHD), myocardial infarction (MI), and angina pectoris.

## B.  MYOCARDIAL INFARCTION

Myocardial infarction (MI) is caused by a sudden deficiency of oxygenated blood to the heart muscle. Symptoms include shortness of breath, perspiration, severe chest pain, and cyanosis. When dental treatment is given to patients who have previously suffered an MI, fear and anxiety must be diminished. Steps that can be taken include administering nitrous oxide sedation, decreasing the length of appointments (no more than 60 minutes), and administering intravenous sedation, with permission of the patient's physician. In general, systemically released epinephrine, which is produced by the body as a reaction to anxiety, is more dangerous than a properly given anesthetic with 1/100,000 concentration of epinephrine. The dentist treating a patient who has suffered an MI should consult with the patient's physician about choice of anesthesia.

## C.  ANGINA PECTORIS

Angina pectoris is a painful condition resulting from a transient deficiency of oxygenated blood supply to the heart. Symptoms include severe, constricting chest pain, anxiety, perspiration, and increased blood pressure. The pain can be caused by exertion or excitement. Treatment includes administering oxygen to assist labored breathing and changing the patient to an upright chair position. Nitroglycerin, a fast-acting drug, is given for relief. Nitroglycerin acts as a **vasodilator,** which causes the blood vessels to relax and dilate. ◀ Consultation with the patient's physician is suggested before dental treatment, and each patient should have nitroglycerin emergency medication readily available and accessible before the dental procedure begins.

## D.  CHEST PAIN

Chest pain that may or may not be caused by a cardiac emergency is managed by stopping dental treatment, shifting the patient to a comfortable position, and administering oxygen, if necessary. If the pain does not subside, the patient may be suffering from a serious cardiac disorder. Medical assistance should be summoned immediately. If a patient loses consciousness, basic life support techniques should be started. These include placing the patient in a supine position, maintaining the airway, checking the pulse, and administering artificial respiration or oxygen, if necessary. If the pulse disappears, CPR should be started immediately. CPR is a technique that supplements artificial respiration with manual artificial circulation. Special training is required before CPR should be attempted. An individual who lacks the required CPR skills may actually cause injury to the patient.

## Summary

- Emergency support telephone numbers must be posted conveniently near each office telephone.
- Basic components of an emergency kit include an oxygen delivery system, noninjectable drugs, and injectable drugs.
- Respiratory failure can occur from obstruction of the airway, hyperventilation, bronchial asthma, heart failure, or acute pulmonary edema.
- Treat hyperventilation by having the patient breathe into a paper bag to increase $CO_2$ blood level.
- Cyanosis may occur in a severe attack of bronchial asthma.
- Administer oxygen and seat patient in upright position if signs of acute heart failure are present. Summon medical assistance.
- CPR requires special training and should be attempted only by individuals with these skills.
- The objective of artificial respiration is to maintain an open airway and mechanically breathe for the victim.
- Patients suffering from congestive heart failure (CHF) cannot lie in a supine position due to fluid retention in the lungs.
- Myocardial infarction is caused by a sudden deficiency of oxygenated blood to the heart muscle.
- Nitroglycerin, a fast-acting vasodilator, is given for relief of angina pectoris.
- If a patient loses consciousness, basic life support techniques should be started.

## IX. SHOCK

**Shock**

Shock occurs when the body's vital functions reach a depressed state.
Anaphylactic shock—Sudden allergic reaction.
Insulin shock—Hypoglycemia or low blood sugar.

**Shock** occurs when the body's vital functions reach a depressed state. It can be caused by trauma, infection, heart attack, smoke, burns, poisoning, lack of oxygen, or obstruction or injury to the air passage. Shock can be exacerbated by abnormal changes in the body temperature, pain, rough handling, and delay in treatment. In some cases, it can be life threatening.

There are two stages of shock. In the early stage, the skin may be pale and cold or the individual may be weak and exhibit a rapid pulse. Breathing may be shallow or deep and irregular, and nausea, vomiting, or anxiety may occur. In the late stage, shock symptoms become more acute. The person becomes unresponsive, and the eyes appear vacant, with dilated pupils. Blood pressure falls and temperature decreases. Loss of consciousness or even death can occur.

Treating shock in a dental office requires that those rendering first aid be skilled in the use of a sphygmomanometer, stethoscope, and oxygen delivery system and knowledgeable about the principles of cardiac and respiratory resuscitation. If it is suspected that a patient is in shock, the following steps should be taken: stop dental treatment, record vital signs, place the patient in a supine position, keep the patient comfortable at room temperature, maintain airway, provide oxygen, and immediately summon medical assistance.

Some causes of shock in patients during dental treatment are cardiogenic shock from acute heart failure, hematogenic shock from hemorrhage, and neurogenic shock from neurologic or psychologic disorders.

## A.  ANAPHYLACTIC SHOCK

Anaphylaxis is a sudden allergic reaction to exposure to an allergen in the body. The allergen may be a certain type of food or particular medication that causes an immediate, potentially life-threatening emergency. The rapid release of histamines by the body may cause severe swelling and edema. Of particular concern is the swelling of the bronchi and trachea. If the airway is blocked, the patient may begin to show signs of **cyanosis,** a bluish skin tone due to lack ◄ of oxygen. Management of the emergency requires administration of epinephrine in the arm or thigh and oxygen, if possible, to assist labored breathing. Vital signs should be closely monitored, and the patient's physician should be consulted, if necessary. Careful review of the patient's medical history for any known **allergy** (hyper- ◄ sensitivity to a substance) should be performed prior to dental treatment.

## B.  INSULIN SHOCK

Diabetes is a metabolic disorder of the body. Hypoglycemia, or insulin shock, may occur when there is too much insulin in the body and the blood sugar level is low. This disorder can occur if the patient forgets to eat on time after taking the insulin medication or from overexertion. Symptoms include headache, feelings of dizziness (vertigo), general weakness, clammy skin, and confusion. Management of this condition includes administering something sweet to eat, such as sugar, candy, or orange juice. If necessary, the patient's physician should be consulted for follow-up treatment.

## X.  SYNCOPE

**Syncope,** or fainting, is a transient loss of consciousness that can oc- ◄ cur during any phase of dental treatment. Symptoms include pallor, discomfort, weakness, perspiration, cold and clammy skin, and temporary loss of consciousness. It is usually a harmless situation, but all loss of consciousness must be regarded as potentially life-threatening. Contributing factors include anxiety, fear, emotional stress, exhaustion, and poor physical condition. The patient should be placed in a **Trendelenburg** position, in which the feet are slightly elevated ◄ in relation to the head. The airway should be established, and tight clothing should be loosened. Spirits of ammonia and oxygen (portable unit 100% $O_2$ delivery system) may be administered.

| Syncope |
| --- |
| Patient will feel faint. Check vitals. Place patient in Trendelenburg position with feet elevated. Administer spirits of ammonia and $O_2$ if necessary. |

## XI.  POSTURAL HYPOTENSION

Postural hypotension, also known as orthostatic hypotension, occurs when the body's autonomic nervous system is unable to compensate for the changes in blood pressure resulting from rapid changes in body position. Patients who remain in a supine position for a long period of time and are suddenly placed in an upright position may experience postural hypotension. Symptoms include a sudden drop in blood pressure and lightheadedness. Treatment includes placing the patient in a supine position, maintaining the airway, administer-

| Postural Hypotension |
| --- |
| Caused by rapid change in body position. Place patient in supine position and administer $O_2$ if necessary. Monitor vital signs. |

ing oxygen, if necessary, and slowly changing the patient's position before dismissal.

## XII. CEREBROVASCULAR ACCIDENT

A cerebrovascular accident (CVA or stroke) is a neurologic disorder in the brain caused by a vascular insufficiency resulting from hemorrhage or formation of blood clots that interfere with or stop oxygenated blood flow. Transient ischemia attacks (TIA) are minor strokes that last for minutes or hours and may include symptoms of headache, confusion, difficulty in speech, dizziness, ringing in the ears, weakness in arms and legs, and personality changes. TIAs may be warning for major CVAs.

If a patient undergoing dental treatment suffers a TIA, the procedure should be stopped, and medical attention should be suggested to the patient as soon as possible. Signs and symptoms of major strokes may include unconsciousness, paralysis or weakness of upper or lower extremities, difficulty in breathing, and a problem with speech. If a patient suffers a major stroke, signs and symptoms should be managed, and medical assistance should be summoned immediately. It may be necessary to supply life support, including CPR.

## XIII. CONVULSIVE DISORDERS

### Convulsive Disorders

Petit mal—Mild seizures
Grand mal—Severe seizures

Epilepsy is a chronic disease characterized by involuntary muscle contractions **(convulsions).** These episodes may be mild convulsions (petit mal), symptomized by twitching muscles and momentary disorientation, or more severe seizures (grand mal), including symptoms of muscle spasms, thrashing, foaming or drooling at the mouth, rolling eyes, and a loss of consciousness. Management of grand mal seizures includes placing the patient in a supine position with the head tilted to the side so that saliva and and vomitus exit, thus decreasing the chance of aspiration of fluids into the lungs. Loosening tight clothing, maintaining an open airway, and removing objects that might injure a thrashing patient are other recommended procedures. Do not attempt to force any object into the patient's mouth during a convulsion. Medical assistance may be necessary. The oral health care delivery team should be supportive of the patient's emotional needs.

## XIV. CHOKING

Choking may occur from certain dental materials or dental prostheses. The patient should be placed in a comfortable position and encouraged to cough in order to remove the obstruction. If a conscious patient is in severe distress, stand behind the patient and deliver abdominal thrusts until the obstruction is cleared. This is also known as the Heimlich maneuver (Fig. 8–4). If the choking is not relieved by these measures, medical emergency assistance should be sought as soon as possible. If breathing stops, basic life support measures must be started immediately. A chest thrust is recommended for patients who are obese or in advanced pregnancy.

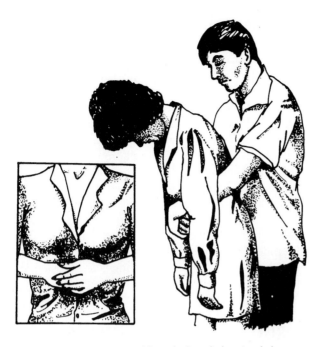

Figure 8–4.  Position of hands for abdominal thrusts.

## XV.   METABOLIC DISORDERS

### A.  *DIABETES MELLITUS*

Diabetes mellitus is a chronic disease associated with carbohydrate, fat, and protein metabolism. The diabetic patient in the dental office can present several types of emergencies, including those related to the vascular consequences of the disease (MI, angina, and stroke). Most emergencies, however, will be caused by insulin therapy, resulting in a blood sugar level that is either too high or too low.

If a patient suffers from hyperglycemia as a result of above normal levels of blood sugar, he or she may suffer abdominal pain, nausea or vomiting, and intense thirst. The breath might have an acetone odor, and the skin may appear dry and flushed. Medical assistance should be summoned immediately.

An emergency associated with diabetes mellitus can be avoided by following general rules. Diabetic patients should be treated in the morning and questioned to determine whether diet and insulin therapy are properly coordinated.

### B.  *HYPERTHYROIDISM*

Hyperthyroidism is a disease caused by excessive production of thyroid hormones. In general, patients with this problem have an increased basal metabolic rate that may be manifested in rapid heart rate, sweating, headache, increased blood pressure, and anxiety. In addition, there might be an increase in cardiac problems. If these symptoms appear, dental treatment should be stopped, and a medical consultation should be suggested. Additionally, local anesthesia containing epinephrine should never be given to such patients, since it may intensify the condition.

### Diabetic Acidosis

Diabetic acidosis or hyperglycemia is caused by above normal levels of blood sugar.

## XVI.  BLEEDING DISORDERS

Simple bleeding can occur as a result of certain dental procedures. Careful medical histories should be elicited so the doctor can be aware of any conditions that might predispose a patient to prolonged bleeding. There are three sources of bleeding: arterial bleeding, in which the blood is bright red and spurting, venous bleeding, in which the blood is darker and flows continuously, and capillary bleeding, in which the blood is bright red and flows slowly and steadily. Most bleeding can be controlled by isolating the area and applying pressure as directly as possible. The patient should be watched carefully for signs of shock. If bleeding does not subside with pressure, the area should be anesthetized in preparation for further treatment. If the bleeding is of capillary origin, sponges impregnated with epinephrine hydrochloride (1/1000) or absorbable gelatin sponges can be packed in the bleeding site. Closing the wound tightly with sutures also can stop the bleeding.

## XVII.  DRUG-INDUCED EMERGENCIES

Complications may arise from local anesthesia. Allergic reactions have decreased dramatically with the introduction of amide anesthesia. (The traditional anesthesia is of the ester type.) Some reactions do occur, however, and may range from simple dermatitis to fatal anaphylactic shock. Often these reactions occur in response to preservatives or other ingredients in the anesthetic solution. The most common reaction from local anesthesia is tachycardia, or rapid

TABLE 8–2.  DOSAGE GUIDELINES FOR LOCAL ANESTHETIC AGENTS

| DRUG | CLASS | MAXIMUM SAFE DOSAGE |
|---|---|---|
| Lidocaine (Xylocaine) 2% without epinephrine | Amide | 4.4 mg/kg up to 300 mg (8.3 carpules) |
| Lidocaine (Xylocaine) 2% with epinephrine | Amide | 6.6 mg/kg up to 500 mg (13.8 carpules) |
| Mepivicaine (Carbocaine) 3% without vasoconstrictor | Amide | 270 mg (5 carpules) |
| Mepivicaine (Carbocaine) 2% with 1:20,000 Neocobefrin | Amide | 180 mg (5 carpules) |
| Prilocaine (Citanest forte) with 1:20,000 epinephrine | Amide | 8 mg/kg up to 600 mg (8 carpules) |
| Propoxycaine (Ravocaine) 0.4% and Procaine (Novocaine) 2% with 1:30,000 levophed | Ester | The manufacturer recommends average dose of 1.8 mL, although this dose may be doubled if necessary |

*Note:* The maximum recommended dosage without significant effect at any one time is 0.2 mg which is approximately equivalent to 10 carpules of 1:100,000. Cardiac patients should always be evaluated closely with regard to the use of epinephrine. Dosage is defined as a body mass-dependent variable. Guidelines based on healthy adult male weighing approximately 70 kg.

heart beat, caused by an exogenous release of epinephrine. Dental treatment should be stopped, and the patient should be made comfortable in a supine position until symptoms subside.

An overdose of anesthetic can cause convulsive reactions or even death (Table 8–2). Factors that can affect the dosage are age (younger and older patients are more sensitive), low body weight, impaired liver and kidney function, or a metabolic disorder. Since an overdose of anesthetic is preventable, it is incumbent on the dentist to evaluate each patient for correct dosage. If the patient has a reaction to the anesthetic, dental treatment should be stopped, basic life support steps should be undertaken, and emergency medical assistance should be summoned as quickly as possible, if needed.

## Summary

- Shock occurs when the body's vital functions reach a depressed state.
- Early signs and symptoms of shock include rapid pulse, pale or cold skin, and weakness.
- Anaphylaxis is a sudden allergic reaction.
- Insulin shock (hypoglycemia) may occur when there is too much insulin in the body and the blood sugar level is low.
- When treating syncope, place patient in a Trendelenburg position.
- Patients may experience postural hypotension if suddenly placed in an upright position.
- Stroke or cerebrovascular accident (CVA) is a neurologic disorder in the brain caused by a vascular insufficiency.
- Epilepsy is a chronic disease characterized by convulsion-like seizures.
- Choking victims may be treated by administering abdominal thrusts.
- The hyperglycemic patient experiences above normal levels of blood sugar. The breath may have an acetone odor.
- Local anesthesia containing epinephrine should not be given to patients who have hyperthyroidism.
- Patients who experience clotting problems or prolonged bleeding should be closely monitored for possible signs of shock.
- Evaluate each patient for correct anesthetic dosage. Anesthetic overdose can cause convulsive reactions or even death.

# Review Questions

1. Discuss the importance of collecting current information about a patient's medical and dental health history.

2. With respect to medical disorders, explain how the health history can provide critical information prior to performing dental procedures.

3. Why are a patient's vital signs taken prior to treatment?

4. Define blood pressure and explain how blood pressure is measured.

5. Identify the average range of blood pressure for an adult.

6. Identify the average pulse rate for adult males.

7. Identify the average respiration rate for adults.

8. What is the average measurement for body temperature?

9. Explain how the dental office can be prepared for an emergency. Your answer should include: emergency equipment, the emergency kit, and training of office personnel.

10. Describe what can occur to the body as a result of a respiratory emergency.

11. List the symptoms and treatment for hyperventilation.

12. What are the symptoms of a bronchial asthma attack?

13. Review the steps in administering artificial respiration if the patient has a pulse.

14. Review the steps in administering artificial respiration if there is a severe injury to the mouth.

15. What preventative steps can be taken to treat a dental patient who has a history of myocardial infarction?

16. Describe how to treat the dental patient who is experiencing an angina attack.

17. What immediate steps must be initiated if a medical emergency arises in which the patient has lost consciousness?

18. Describe the stages of shock. Your answer should include signs and symptoms.

19. Describe how to treat an anaphylactic shock emergency.

20. Explain the medical emergency procedure for treating a patient who may be in insulin shock.

21. Discuss the signs and symptoms of syncope and the methods of treating this type of medical emergency.

22. How can postural hypotension be prevented?

23. What is the treatment for a medical emergency involving postural hypotension?

24. Describe the signs and symptoms of a transient ischemia attack (TIA).

25. Explain the medical emergency procedures for treating a stroke victim.

26. Distinguish between a petit mal and grand mal seizure.

27. Explain the medical emergency steps for treating an epileptic convulsive seizure.

28. What is meant by the Heimlich maneuver? Why is the Heimlich maneuver performed?

29. Discuss the signs and symptoms of a patient experiencing hyperglycemia.

30. Indicate the best time of day to treat diabetic patients.

31. Explain why local anesthesia containing epinephrine should not be given to patients who have a history of hyperthyroidism.

32. Discuss the three sources of bleeding.

33. Describe alternative methods of controlling bleeding if direct pressure applications are not effective in stopping the flow of blood.

34. How can an overdose of local anesthesia be avoided?

# Occupational Safety

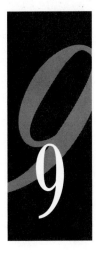

## Key Terms ◀

BLOODBORNE PATHOGEN
STANDARD

BIOHAZARD

ENGINEERING CONTROLS

EXPOSURE INCIDENT

EYEWASH STATION

HAZARD COMMUNICATION
STANDARD

HEPATITIS-B VIRUS

HUMAN IMMUNODEFICIENCY
VIRUS

MATERIAL SAFETY DATA SHEET

OFFICE SAFETY COORDINATOR

OSHA

SOURCE INDIVIDUAL

WORK PRACTICE CONTROLS

WRITTEN EXPOSURE CONTROL
PLAN

WRITTEN HAZARD COMMUNICA-
TION PROGRAM

## I. INTRODUCTION

Regulatory compliance issues affecting occupational and office safety
for all dental health care workers have mandated the implementation
of strict protocols over infection control procedures and the management of hazardous materials in the dental office. **OSHA** (Occupa- ◀
tional Safety and Health Administration), a division of the United
States Department of Labor, is the regulatory body which oversees
the protection of all workers from physical, chemical, or infectious
hazards in the work place.

The dental assistant is often delegated the responsibility of **of- ◀
fice safety coordinator.** Coordination includes staff training in
aseptic techniques and safe handling of hazardous materials. The of-

fice safety coordinator oversees required OSHA office recordkeeping, biohazard labeling, and maintenance of an office infection control manual. This chapter will present an overview of the OSHA Bloodborne Pathogen Standard and Hazard Communication Standard.

## II.  BLOODBORNE PATHOGEN STANDARD

▶ The **Bloodborne Pathogen Standard** was initiated to provide protection to all health care workers who come in contact with bloodborne pathogens. During infection, bloodborne pathogens can exist in the blood or other body fluid tissues such as saliva. The likelihood of disease transmission (spreading a disease from one person to another by contact with infectious fluids) is increased in dentistry.

▶ **Hepatitis B virus** (HBV) and **human immunodeficiency virus** (HIV) are caused by viruses that may be found in blood or other body fluids. The potential for occupational exposure by health care workers to these infectious pathogens can be prevented by complying with OSHA's bloodborne pathogen standard.

Key requirements of OSHA's bloodborne pathogen standard include a wide combination of provisions and controls which address a number of specific practices for the workplace. The following requirements highlight key components of OSHA's bloodborne pathogen standard.

- Personal protective equipment (PPE)
- Establishment of engineering/work practice controls
- Housekeeping
- Waste handling
- Employee medical records/vaccination records
- Laundering
- Written exposure control plan

---

**OSHA Requirements: Occupational Exposure to Bloodborne Pathogen Standard**

1. Personal protective equipment
2. Engineering/work practice controls
3. Housekeeping
4. Waste handling
5. Employee medical records/vaccination
6. Laundering
7. Written exposure control plan

---

**Personal Protective Equipment**

Face shield/face mask
Eyewear
Clinic jacket/lab coat
Disposable gloves
Utility gloves
Resuscitation bags/mouthpieces

---

## III.  CONTROLLING OCCUPATIONAL EXPOSURE TO BLOODBORNE PATHOGENS

Personal protective equipment is comprised of specialized clothing or equipment worn by employees to protect themselves from exposure to blood or other potentially infectious materials. Personal protective equipment must not allow blood or other potentially infectious materials to pass through to clothing, skin, or mucous membranes.

*Personal protective equipment includes the following:*

- *Face protection:* A chin-length face shield or a combination of mask with eye protection should be used. A mask must be worn with a face shield.
- *Eye protection:* Goggles or eye glasses with solid side shields or face shields can provide adequate eye protection.
- *Clinic jackets, lab coats, gowns:* Protective clothing and equipment must be removed immediately, or as soon as feasible, when penetrated by blood or other infectious materials, and prior to leaving the work area.
- *Gloves:* Gloves must be worn when it is anticipated that an employee will make hand contact with blood or saliva during

procedures; when performing vascular access procedures; or when handling instruments, materials, and surfaces that are contaminated. Disposable gloves must be replaced upon the completion of the dental procedure or if torn or punctured during the procedure. Disposable gloves must not be reused. Utility gloves used for cleanup may be decontaminated for reuse, but must be discarded if they are deteriorated or fail to function as barrier.

- *Resuscitation bags, mouthpieces, and pocket masks:* These ventilation devices minimize the need for mouth-to-mouth resuscitation.

Contaminated PPE must be placed in an appropriately designated area or container for storing, washing, decontaminating or discarding. Contaminated laundry must be placed in a red bag or bag with a biohazard label.

## IV.   ENGINEERING & WORK PRACTICE CONTROLS

> **Engineering Controls**
>
> Engineering controls isolate or remove the hazard from the employee (eg, rubber dam, sharps container)

Engineering and work practice controls are the primary methods used to control the transmission of HBV and HIV in the dental setting. Personal protective clothing and equipment are also necessary when occupational exposure to bloodborne pathogens remains even after instituting these controls.

As they apply to the dental operatory, **engineering controls** ◄ isolate or remove the hazard from employees. Rubber dams, high speed evacuators, and special containers for contaminated sharp instruments are examples of engineering controls.

Engineering controls must be examined and maintained, or replaced, on a scheduled basis. These engineering controls are used in combination with work practice controls.

**Work practice controls** reduce the likelihood of exposure by ◄ altering the manner in which the task is performed. All procedures must be performed in such a manner as to minimize splashing, spraying, spattering, and generating droplets of blood or other potentially infectious materials.

> **Work Practice Controls**
>
> Work practice controls alter the manner in which the task is performed (eg, prohibiting bending of contaminated needles)

Work practice control requirements include the following:

- Washing hands immediately, or as soon as feasible, after skin contact with blood or other potentially infectious materials and after removing gloves or other personal protective equipment.
- Flushing mucous membranes immediately, or as soon as feasible, if they are splashed with blood or other potentially infectious materials.
- Prohibiting recapping, bending, or removing contaminated needles from syringes, unless required by the dental or medical procedure. If this is the case, recapping must be done by mechanical means, such as mechanical recapper, or using a one-handed (scoop) technique. Recapping is permitted when administering multiple injections of local anesthesia.
- Eliminating the shearing and breaking of contaminated needles.
- Discarding contaminated needles and disposable sharps in containers that are closable, puncture-resistant, leakproof, and colored red or labeled with the biohazard symbol. Containers

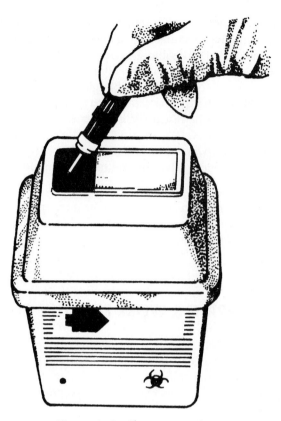

Figure 9–1. Sharps container.

must be easily accessible, maintained upright, and not allowed to overfill. (Fig. 9–1)

- Placing contaminated, reusable, sharp instruments in containers that are puncture resistant, leakproof, and colored red or
  labeled with the biohazard symbol until properly processed.
  Reusable sharps must not be stored or processed in such a
  way that employees are required to reach by hand into the
  container to retrieve the instruments.
- Prohibiting eating, drinking, smoking, applying cosmetics, and
  handling contact lenses in areas where there is occupational
  exposure, such as in a dental operatory or reprocessing areas.
- Eliminating the storage of food and drink in refrigerators, cabinets, shelves, or countertops where blood or other potentially infectious materials are present.
- Storing, transporting, or shipping blood or other potentially
  infectious materials such as extracted teeth, tissue, and impressions that have not been decontaminated in containers
  that are closed, prevent leakage, and are colored red or affixed with the biohazard label.

## V.   HOUSEKEEPING

Work surfaces, equipment, and other reusable items must be decontaminated with disinfectant upon completion of procedures when
contamination occurs through splashes, spills, or other contact with
blood and other potentially infectious materials.

If surfaces, equipment, and other items (such as light handles or trays) have been protected with coverings (such as plastic wrap or foil), these materials must be replaced when contaminated or at the end of the workshift.

Broken glass that may be contaminated may be cleaned up with a brush or tongs; but never picked up with hands, even if gloves are worn.

Equipment that has been in contact with blood or other potentially infectious materials and is to be either serviced on-site or shipped out of the facility for maintenance or other service, must be decontaminated to the extent feasible or labeled as a biohazard, indicating which parts were not decontaminated.

## VI.  WASTE HANDLING

*Waste removed from the facility may be regulated by a combination of local, state, and federal laws.* To comply with the bloodborne pathogens standard, special precautions are necessary when disposing of *contaminated sharps and other regulated waste.*

Contaminated disposable sharps must be placed in containers that are closable, puncture resistant, leakproof, and colored red or labeled with the **biohazard** symbol. Other regulated waste generated from dental procedures also must be contained in closable bags or containers that prevent leakage and are colored red or labeled with the biohazard symbol. (Fig. 9–2)

A secondary container is necessary for containers that are contaminated on the outside. The secondary container must also be closable, prevent leakage, and be color-coded or labeled.

Regulated waste is defined as liquid or semi-liquid blood or other potentially infectious materials; items contaminated with blood or other potentially infectious materials that would release these substances in a liquid or semi-liquid state if compressed; items that are caked with dried blood or other potentially infectious materials and are capable of releasing these materials during handling; contaminated sharps; and pathological and microbiological wastes containing blood or other potentially infectious materials.

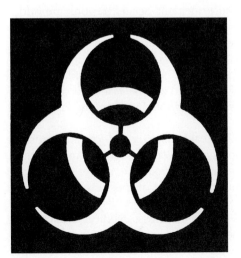

Figure 9–2.  Biohazard symbol.

## Summary

■ OSHA is a regulatory body that oversees the protection of all workers from physical, chemical, or infectious hazards in the workplace.

■ HBV and HIV are caused by viruses which may be found in blood or other body fluids.

■ Personal protective equipment is specialized clothing or equipment worn by employees to protect themselves from exposure to blood.

■ Personal protective equipment includes resuscitation bags, mouthpieces, and pocket masks used for mouth-to-mouth resuscitation.

■ Engineering controls include special containers for contaminated sharp instruments.

■ Work practice controls alter the manner in which a task is performed.

■ All surfaces, equipment, and other reusable items must be decontaminated with a disinfectant when contamination occurs through splashes, spills, or other contact with blood or a potentially infectious material.

■ Contaminated disposable sharps must be placed in containers that are closable, puncture resistant, leakproof, and are colored red or labeled with the biohazard symbol.

■ Compliance of local, state, and federal laws is necessary for the removal of regulated waste.

## VII.  RECORDKEEPING—MEDICAL & TRAINING RECORDS

A medical record must be established for each employee with occupational exposure. This record is confidential and separate from other personnel records. This record may be kept on-site or may be retained by the health care professional who provides services to the dental health care employees. The medical record contains the hepatitis B vaccination status, including the dates of the hepatitis B vaccination and the written opinion of the health care professional regarding the hepatitis B vaccination.

If an occupational exposure incident occurs, reports are added to the medical record to document the incident and the results of testing following the incident, as well as the written opinion of the health care professional. The medical record also must indicate what documents have been provided to the health care provider. Medical records must be maintained 30 years past the last date of employment of the employee. *The confidentiality of medical records must be emphasized.*

Training records document each training session and must be kept by the employer for three years. Training records must include the date of the training, a content outline, the trainer's name and qualifications, and names and job titles of all persons attending the training sessions.

If the employer ceases to do business, medical and training records are transferred to the successor employer. Training records must be available to employees or employee representatives upon request. Medical records can be obtained by the employee or anyone having the employee's written consent. Additional recordkeeping is required for employers with eleven or more employees.

## VIII.   VACCINATION—HEPATITIS B

The hepatitis B vaccination must be made available within ten working days of initial assignment to every employee whose job classification or tasks result in occupational exposure. Employees who choose to decline the vaccination for hepatitis B must sign a statement to that effect. The employee who continues to be at occupational risk for hepatitis B may request from their employer to obtain the hepatitis B vaccination at a later date.

## IX.   LAUNDRY

Contaminated laundry should be handled as little as possible with minimum agitation. Laundering contaminated articles, including employee clinic jackets and lab coats used as PPE, is the responsibility of the employer. This can be accomplished through the use of a washer and dryer in a designated area on-site, or a commercial laundry that processes contaminated laundry.

Contaminated laundry must be placed in bags or containers that are red or are marked with the biohazard symbol. If the office uses Universal Precautions in handling all soiled laundry, alternative labeling is permitted, provided that all employees are appropriately trained to recognize that the bags contain contaminated laundry.

If the laundry is sent off site for cleaning, it must be in bags or containers that are clearly marked with the biohazard symbol. Bags or containers must prevent leakage and soak-through when contaminated laundry is wet. Gloves and other appropriate personal protective equipment must always be worn when handling contaminated laundry.

## X.   EXPOSURE CONTROL PLAN

A **written exposure control plan** that provides documentation of ◀
the following key elements is required:

- Identification of job classifications and tasks where there is exposure to blood and other potentially infectious materials.
- A schedule of how and when the provisions of the standard will be implemented, including schedules and methods for communication of hazards to employees, hepatitis B vaccination and post-exposure evaluation and followup, recordkeeping and implementation of the methods of compliance such as engineering and work practice controls, PPE, housekeeping, laundry, etc.
- *Procedures for evaluating the circumstances of an exposure incident.*
- The written exposure control plan must be accessible to employees and must be updated at least annually and when alterations in procedures create new occupational exposure.

## XI. EXPOSURE INCIDENT FOLLOW-UP

▶ An **exposure incident** is a specific eye, mouth, other mucous membrane, non-intact skin, or parenteral contact with blood or other potentially infectious materials that results from the performance of an employee's duties.

*An example of an exposure incident would include a puncture from a contaminated sharp instrument.* If injury by a contaminated instrument occurs, or blood contacts the skin, mucous membranes, nose, or mouth, the exposed area must be immediately cleaned by washing contaminated skin with soap and water. Mucous membranes should be irrigated with sterile normal saline. Eyes should be washed at an eyewash station with plain water.

Employees should immediately report exposure incidents to their employer to initiate a timely follow-up process by a health care professional. This report initiates the procedure for a prompt request for evaluation of the source individual's HBV and HIV status (Figs. 9–3, 9–4).

▶ **"Source individual"** is any patient whose blood or body fluids are the source of an exposure incident to the employee. Testing the source individual's blood cannot be done in most states without written consent. The results of the source individual's blood tests are confidential and should be directed only to the attending health care professional.

As soon as possible, test results of the source individual's blood must be made available to the exposed employee through consultation with the health care professional.

The employee who has had an exposure incident must be directed to a health care professional. *The employer must provide the health care professional with a copy of the following:*

- Bloodborne pathogens standard
- Description of employee's job duties relative to the incident
- Incident report
- Route(s) of exposure
- Source individual's blood test results, if available
- Employee medical records/vaccination status

At that time, a baseline blood test to establish the employee's HIV and HBV status will be drawn, if the employee consents. The employee has the right to decline testing or to delay HIV testing for up to 90 days. During this time, the health care professional must preserve the employee's blood sample.

Following post-exposure evaluation, the health care professional will provide a written opinion to the employer. The written opinion is limited to a statement that the employee has been informed of the results of the evaluation, and told of the need, if any, for further evaluation or treatment. *All other findings are confidential.* The employer must provide a copy of the written opinion to the employee within 15 days of the evaluation.

If the employee requires further medical attention, the information must be entered in the employee medical record. This medical record is confidential and is separate from other personnel records. Medical records are to be maintained for the term of employment plus an additional thirty years.

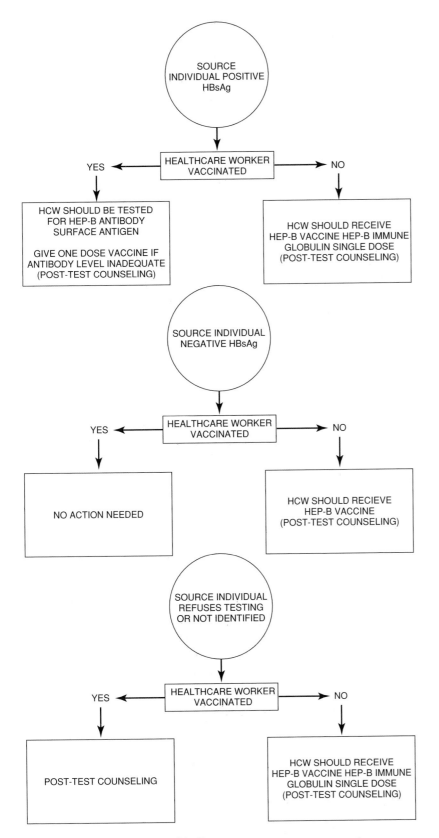

Figure 9–3.  Hepatitis-B post exposure management.

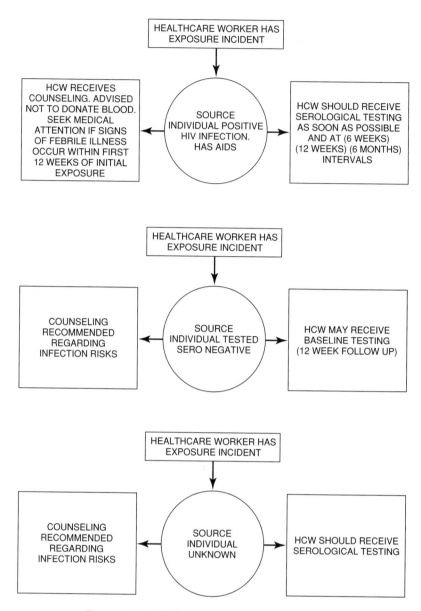

Figure 9–4. HIV post exposure management.

# XII.   EMPLOYEE COMMUNICATION PROGRAM

Training for dental employees regarding the bloodborne pathogen standard must be provided at no cost to the employee and during working hours. Training is also required for new employees at the time of initial assignment of tasks with occupational exposure or when job tasks change, causing a change in occupational exposure. Annual retraining for all affected employees must be provided.

*During training sessions, the following information must be communicated and explained to the employee by the office safety program coordinator:*

- Copy of the bloodborne pathogen standard and explanation of content
- Epidemiology and symptoms of bloodborne diseases

- Modes of transmission of bloodborne pathogens
- Employee's written exposure control plan and how to obtain a copy
- How to recognize an occupational exposure
- Methods to control occupational transmission of bloodborne pathogens
- Personal protective equipment (PPE)
- Hepatitis B vaccine and vaccination information
- Emergencies involving blood and other potentially infectious materials
- Reporting mechanism for exposure incidents
- Post-exposure evaluation and follow-up
- Explanation of labels, signs, and markings for contaminated materials
- Discussion of preventive measures, including engineering and safe work practice controls, housekeeping measures, universal precautions
- Opportunity for questions and answers

## Summary

- A medical record must be established for each employee with occupational exposure.
- Training records must be kept by the employer for three years.
- The hepatitis B vaccination must be made available to every employee within 10 working days of initial assignment.
- Contaminated laundry should be handled as little as possible with minimum agitation.
- Laundry that is sent off-site for cleaning must be in bags or containers that are clearly marked with the biohazard symbol.
- Written exposure control plan must include identification of job classifications and tasks.
- Written exposure control plan must be accessible to employees and updated at least annually.
- A puncture from a contaminated sharp instrument is an example of an exposure incident.
- Wash eyes, if contaminated, at eyewash station with plain water.
- Exposure incidents should be reported to the employer immediately.
- "Source individual" is any patient whose blood or body fluids are the source of an exposure incident to the employee.
- Training of dental employees regarding the bloodborne pathogen standard must be provided on an annual basis.

## XIII.  HAZARD COMMUNICATION STANDARD

OSHA's **Hazard Communication Standard** was initiated to protect all workers who may come in contact with potential injuries and illnesses from exposure to hazardous chemicals in the workplace. The Hazard Communication Standard covers both physical hazards (such as flammability) and health hazards (such as irritation, lung damage, and cancer).

The standard was implemented in health care settings to ensure that all employees who handle, use, and store hazardous materials

**OSHA Requirements: Hazard Communication Standard**

1. Material Safety Data Sheets (MSDS)
2. Labeling
3. Record keeping
4. Written hazard communication program

receive information from their employers on the hazards of these chemicals. Chemical information to be conveyed to the employee includes product label warnings, product handling and disposal methods, and use of personal protective devices for safer product handling.

The information concerning the hazards of workplace chemicals is to be transmitted directly to the employee by the employer through training sessions and a *written hazard communication program.*

Additional key components of OSHA's hazard communication standard include:

- Material Safety Data Sheets (MSDS)
- Labeling of hazardous chemicals
- Recordkeeping of training sessions
- Posting of OSHA Poster Form 2203

## XIV.   MATERIAL SAFETY DATA SHEETS

▶ Chemical manufacturers and importers must develop a **material safety data sheet** (MSDS) for each hazardous chemical they produce or import and must provide the MSDS automatically at the time of the initial shipment of a hazardous chemical to a downstream distributor or user. Distributors must also ensure that downstream employers are similarly provided an MSDS.

Each MSDS must be in English and include information regarding the specific chemical identity of the hazardous chemicals involved and the common names. In addition, information must be provided on the physical and chemical characteristics of the hazardous chemical, known acute and chronic health effects and related health information, exposure limits, whether the chemical is considered to be a carcinogen, precautionary measures, emergency and first-aid procedures, and the identification of the organization responsible for preparing the sheet. *The MSDS provides useful chemical information which will assist labeling and development of warning signs.*

Employers must prepare a list of all hazardous chemicals in the workplace. When the list is complete, it should be checked against the collected MSDS that the employer has been sent. If there are hazardous chemicals used for which no MSDS has been received, the employer must write to the supplier, manufacturer, or importer to obtain the missing MSDS.

Copies of the MSDS for hazardous chemicals in a given work site are to be readily accessible to employees in that area. As a source of detailed information on hazards, they must be located close to workers and be readily available to them during each workshift. MSDS sheets may be kept in a binder in a central location or accessed by computer terminals.

MSDS sheets provide detailed information on each hazardous chemical and include the identified chemicals' physical and chemical properties, potential for hazardous effects, and recommendations for appropriate protective measures during exposure.

There is no specified format for the MSDS, but each MSDS must provide at least the following information. (Figure 9–5 is an example of a typical MSDS.)

# MATERIAL SAFETY DATA SHEET

## SECTION I - MATERIAL IDENTIFICATION AND USE

Controlled Product    Yes ☐    No ☑

| | |
|---|---|
| Material Name: Ultra-Etch® 35% and 10% | Product Identification Number: REF/UP 163, 164, 167, 168, 271, 272, 273, 274, 677, and 685. |
| Manufacturer's Name: Ultradent Products, Inc. | Chemical Family: Acids |
| Street Address: 505 West 10200 South | Chemical Formula: 35% - $H_3PO_4$ |
| City: South Jordan    State: Utah    USA | 10% - $H_3PO_4$ |
| Zip: 84095    Emergency Telephone No.: 800-552-5512 | Trade Name and Synonyms: Ultra-Etch® - Enamel and Dentin Etch |
| Chemical Name: Phosphoric Acid | Material Use: Etching of tooth enamel and dentin. |
| Molecular Weight: N/A | |

## SECTION II - HAZARDOUS INGREDIENTS OF MATERIAL

| Hazardous Ingredients | Approximate Concentration % | C.A.S. N.A. or U.N. Numbers | "Exposure limits" | LD50/LC50 Specify Species and Route |
|---|---|---|---|---|
| Phosphoric Acid | 35% | 7664-38-2 | | $LD_{50}$ - oral rat 1530 mg/kg |
| Phosphoric Acid | 10% | 7664-38-2 | | $LD_{50}$ - oral rat 1530 mg/kg |

## SECTION III - PHYSICAL DATA FOR MATERIAL

| | | | | |
|---|---|---|---|---|
| Physical State: Gas ☐  Gel ☑  Solid ☐ | Odor and Appearance: Odorless; Blue (35%), Bright Red (10%) | | Odor Threshold (p.p.m.): N/A | Specific Gravity: 1.32 (35%) 1.12 (10%) |
| Vapor Pressure (mm Hg): N/A | Vapor Density (Air = 1): N/A | Evaporation Rate: N/A | Boiling Point (°C): | Freezing Point (°C): about -1°C |
| Solubility in Water (20° C): 95% | % Volatile (by volume): N/A | pH: < 2 | about 100°C | Coefficient of water/oil distribution: N/A |

## SECTION IV - FIRE AND EXPLOSION HAZARD OF MATERIAL

Flammability: Yes ☐  No ☑    If Yes, under which conditions:

Means of Extinction: N/A

Special Procedures: N/A

| | | |
|---|---|---|
| Flash point (°C) and Method: N/A | Upper explosion limit (% by volume): N/A | Lower explosion limit (% by volume): N/A |
| Auto Ignition Temperature (°C): N/A | | Hazardous Combustion Products: N/A |

| | | | |
|---|---|---|---|
| Explosion Data Sensitivity to Mechanical Impact: N/A | Rate of Burning: N/A | Explosive Power: N/A | Sensitivity to Static Discharge: N/A |

## SECTION V - REACTIVITY DATA

Chemical Stability: Yes ☑  No ☐    If No, under which conditions:

Incompatibility to other substances: Yes ☑  No ☐    If Yes, which ones: Bases (strong), common metals.

Reactivity and under what conditions: Chemical reaction when mixed together with bases, corrosive.

Hazardous Decomposition Products: Oxides of phosphorus.

Material Name/Identifier: Ultra-Etch

**UP® ULTRADENT PRODUCTS, INC.**

Figure 9–5. MSDS sheet. (Courtesy of Ultradent Products, Inc.)

## SECTION VI - TOXICOLOGICAL PROPERTIES OF PRODUCT

| Route of Entry | ☑ Skin Contact | ☐ Skin Absorption | ☑ Eye Contact | ☐ Inhalation Acute | ☐ Inhalation Chronic | ☑ Ingestion |
|---|---|---|---|---|---|---|

**Effects of Acute Exposure to Product**

Skin - may cause skin irritation. Eyes - severe eye irritaion. Ingestion - possible irritation.

**Effects of Chronic Exposure to Product** Skin - mild irritation. Eyes - damage eyes (chronic exposure must be avoided). Ingestion - irritation will occur.

| LD$_{50}$ of Product (Specify Species and Route) | Not established. | Irritancy of Product | Mild | Exposure limits of Product | N/A |
|---|---|---|---|---|---|
| LC$_{50}$ of Product (Specify Species) | N/A | Sensitization to Product | N/A | Synergistic materials | N/A |

☐ Carcinogenicity  ☐ Reproductive effects  ☐ Teratogenicity  ☐ Mutagenicity  N/A

## SECTION VII - PREVENTIVE MEASURES

| Personal Protective Equipment | Protective Eyewear | | |
|---|---|---|---|

| Gloves (Specify) | Rubber | Respiratory (Specify) N/A | Eye (Specify) Protective Plastic. | Footwear (Specify) N/A |
|---|---|---|---|---|

| Clothing (Specify) | N/A | Other (Specify) N/A |
|---|---|---|

**Engineering Controls** (e.g. ventilation, enclosed process, specify) N/A

**Leak and Spill Procedure** Clean up with wet rag. Neutralize with baking soda.

**Waste Disposal** Wipe up and throw in trash.

**Handling Procedures and Equipment** Use gloves and protective eyewear.

**Storage Requirements** Store at room temperature.

**Special Shipping Information** None

## SECTION VIII - FIRST AID MEASURES

**Skin**

Flush with water.

**Eye**

Flush immediately with water. Get medical attention.

**Inhalation** N/A

**Ingestion**

Do not induce vomiting. Give large amounts of water or milk. Take an antacid. Call physician.

**General advice** FOR DENTAL USE ONLY - Use as directed.

## SECTION IX - PREPARATION DATE OF M.S.D.S.

**Additional Information** Only very small dosages are used in dentistry - usually not hazardous.

**Sources Used** Raw Material MSDS and MFG's Knowledge.

| Prepared by: John Tobler, Chemist | Phone Number 800-552-5512 | Date September 7, 1995 |
|---|---|---|

The information and recommendations are taken from sources believed to be accurate; however, Ultradent Products, Inc., makes no warranty with respect to the accuracy of the information or the suitability of the recommendation and assumes no liability to any user thereof. Each user should review these recommendations in the specific context of the intended use and determine whether they are appropriate.

**UP®  ULTRADENT PRODUCTS, INC.**

#10995   R003/020796

Figure 9–5. Continued.

**SECTION I**—Identifies the hazardous chemical's name, generic and scientific, the manufacturer's name, address, and contact phone number, and **product information** and use.

**SECTION II**—Lists **hazardous ingredients** of the material. Includes hazard data such as flammability, exposure limits, and median lethal dose (LD50).

**SECTION III**—Provides information on the **physical hazards** of the material. For example, data may include odor and appearance, vapor pressure, physical state, solubility in water, evaporation rate, pH, boiling point, and freezing point.

**SECTION IV**—Provides data relative to the **fire and explosion hazards** of the chemical. Information listed in this section includes means of extinguishing chemical, flash point, rate of burning, flammability, explosive power, and upper and lower explosive limits.

**SECTION V**—**Reactivity data** is provided to assist in safe handling procedures with the chemical. Lists reactions of chemical when in contact with water, sunlight, acids, bases, and metal piping. Incompatibility and stability properties including **hazardous decomposition properties** are also identified.

**SECTION VI**—**Health hazard data** information is presented, including potential hazards from product absorption, threshold limits, routes of exposure, effects of chronic and acute exposures, toxicity, and carcinogenicity.

**SECTION VII**—Includes precautions for safe handling, **preventive measures,** and waste disposal methods of chemical. **Leak and spill procedures,** including ventilation requirements and personal protective equipment, clean-up substance compatibility, engineering controls, storage requirements, and special shipping information are provided.

**SECTION VIII**—Lists information relative to **respiratory protection,** control measures, and first aid measures.

**SECTION IX**—Highlights **special precautions** of listed product. May include preparation date of MSDS and related health or general safety information.

# XV.  LABELING

Chemical manufacturers, importers, and distributors must be sure that containers of hazardous chemicals leaving the workplace are labeled, tagged, or marked. Requirements include the identity of the hazardous chemical, appropriate hazard warnings, and the name and address of the manufacturer or other responsible party.

In the workplace, the employer is responsible for labeling secondary containers which contain hazardous chemicals, such as Ultrasonic Units, and x-ray wet tanks containing developer and fixer solutions. The container must show hazard warnings appropriate for employee protection.

The hazard warning can be any type of message, words, pictures, or symbols that convey the hazards of the chemical(s) in the container. Labels must be legible, in English (and other languages, if desired), and prominently displayed.

The hazard warning is a brief statement of the hazardous effects of the chemical: for example, "flammable" or "causes lung damage." Labels frequently contain other information, such as precautionary

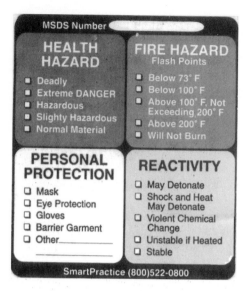

Figure 9–6. Labeling sample. (Courtesy of Smart Practice.)

measures ("Do not use near open flame"), but this information is provided voluntarily and is *not* required by the OSHA rule.

There is no official labeling system that is endorsed by OSHA's regulating body. The office labeling system must be easy to read and all employees must be properly trained to clearly understand the system. If blank containers are used, labels may be photocopied from the original container and applied to the new container. Labels may be color-coded for ease in identification or designated a number rating as to product hazard properties (Fig. 9–6).

# XVI.  TRAINING & EMPLOYEE INFORMATION

Each employee who may be exposed to hazardous chemicals at work must be provided information and training prior to initial assignment to work with a hazardous chemical, and whenever the hazard changes. "Exposure" or "exposed" under the OSHA standard means that "an employee is subjected to a hazardous chemical in the course of employment through any route of entry (inhalation, ingestion, skin contact or absorption, etc) and includes potential (eg, accidental or possible) exposure."

Information and training may be done either by individual chemical, or by categories of hazards (such as flammability or carcinogenicity). Employees will have access to the substance-specific information on the labels and MSDS. Information and training are a critical part of the hazard communication program. Information regarding hazards and protective measures is provided to workers through written labels and material safety data sheets.

# XVII.  WRITTEN HAZARD COMMUNICATION PROGRAM

All workplaces where employees are exposed to hazardous chemicals must have a written plan that describes how the standard will be implemented in that facility. The written program must describe how the

---

## Components Written Hazard Communication Program

1. Prepare inventory of chemicals.
2. Ensure containers are labeled.
3. Obtain MSDS for each chemical. Keep current.
4. Make MSDS available to employees.
5. Conduct training of how to use MSDS.
6. Identify who is delegated to coordinate office Haz. Mat. standard.
7. Training descriptions.
8. Protective measures used to protect employees.
9. Emergency exposure incident reporting.

requirements for labels and other forms of warning, MSDS, and employee information and training, will be met in the workplace. The employer is responsible for the development, implementation, and maintenance of the written hazard communication program. Each employee must be informed as to the location of the written hazard communication program and the collection of MSDS for reference purposes.

The following guidelines will assist in meeting OSHA compliance for an effective **written hazard communication program:** ◀

1. Prepare an inventory of chemicals.
2. Ensure containers are labeled and describe labeling method.
3. Obtain MSDS for each chemical and determine how list will be kept current.
4. Make MSDS available to workers.
5. Conduct training of workers, including how to use MSDS.
6. Identify who is delegated to coordinate office HazMat standard (individual's name and title must be documented).
7. Maintain a description of the procedure used to train employees.
8. Maintain details of the protective measures used to protect employees.
9. Plan emergency exposure incident reporting and follow-up procedures.

## Summary

- The Hazard Communication Standard covers both physical hazards and health hazards.
- Chemical manufacturers and importers must develop a material safety data sheet for each hazardous chemical produced or imported.
- Copies of the MSDS for hazardous chemicals in a given work site are to be readily accessible to all employees.
- The MSDS identifies the chemical's physical and chemical properties, potential for hazardous effects, and recommendations for appropriate protective measures.
- In the workplace, each secondary container must be labeled, tagged, or marked with the identity of hazardous chemical contents.
- Each employee who may be exposed to hazardous chemicals must be provided information and training prior to initial assignment.
- All workplaces where employees are exposed to hazardous chemicals must have a written plan (hazard communication program).

## XVIII. GENERAL DENTAL OFFICE SAFETY GUIDELINES

To minimize hazards in the dental office when handling hazardous chemicals, it is important that all personnel know how to handle accidental spills and have the necessary supplies readily available. All office personnel must be aware of which dental products contain hazardous chemicals and know the hazards associated with the product.

Properly discard chemicals which are no longer used or have

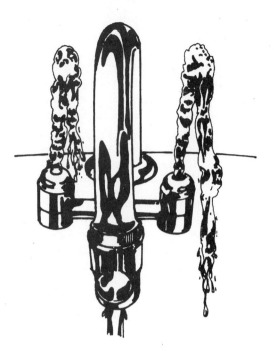

Figure 9–7. Eye wash station.

expired. Order identified hazardous chemical products as needed, and keep stock at a minimum. Use products as directed on the label and follow instructions for proper manipulation. Whenever possible, use protective equipment to minimize chemical contact to skin and hands. Provide proper ventilation to minimize inhalation of chemicals and avoid unnecessary exposure by keeping product containers closed when not in use. Use respiratory protection and NIOSH-approved masks.

Eye protection such as safety glasses and/or goggles is necessary to minimize potential injury to the eyes when working with chemicals and other hazardous materials. Contact lenses do not provide protection to the eyes. If chemicals contact the eye, flush with cold water and seek medical attention as soon as possible. Maintain temperature-regulated **eyewash station** (Fig. 9–7).

Neutralizing agents such as baking soda are effective for certain acid spills. Absorbent materials and nitrile rubber gloves should be part of the office clean up kit. An operational fire extinguisher, portable oxygen resuscitation equipment, and a first aid kit are essential in promoting general dental office safety.

## XIX.  GENERAL PRODUCT SAFETY GUIDELINES

**Acid Etchants:**  Use eye protection. If acid etch solution contacts eyes, flush with cold water and seek medical attention. For etchant spills, use gloves for clean-up and cover spill with baking soda. Etchants include phosphoric acid and citric acid. Acid etch solutions are associated with dental procedures involving placement of sealants, composite resins, and orthodontic brackets.

**Acidulated Fluoride:**  Use eye protection and gloves when handling. Small amounts of phosphoric acid are present in acidulated fluoride. If there has been skin contact, wash affected area with soap and water. If there has been eye contact, flush with cold water and seek medical attention. In case of spill, wipe with sponge.

**Alginate Impression Material:** Alginate powder contains silica, which may be harmful if inhaled in large quantities. Use a mask when working with alginate powders. If there has been eye contact, flush with cold water and seek medical attention. If there has been skin contact, wash affected area with soap and water. Mop up spills.

**BIS-GMA:** BIS-GMA is a possible irritant to skin and eyes. It is found in **dentin bonding systems** and composite resins, and is known as a methacrylate ester. Avoid prolonged exposure or repeated contact when working with BIS-GMA dental materials. Gloves should be worn to clean spills, which should be mopped up with hot, soapy water.

**Bonding Agents for Porcelain:** Small amounts of acetic acid may be found in bonding agents used for repairing broken porcelain or bonding porcelain to another material. In case of skin contact, remove contaminated clothing and flush affected area with water first, then wash with soap and water. If spills occur, sweep up and place absorbent materials in container.

**Dental Stone:** Dental stone contains 100% gypsum, a calcium sulfate hemihydrate. Particles may become airborne and present possible irritation; use of protective eyewear and mask is recommended. Spills may be swept.

**Disinfectants:** Dental disinfectants are very potent and considered hazardous. Gloves and eye protection are recommended. They are mildly toxic by inhalation, and should only be used with proper ventilation. In cases of eye contact, flush with water and seek medical attention. Spills should be soaked up with absorbent materials and placed in a container for disposal.

**Formaldehyde:** Formaldehyde is used in chemical-vapor sterilization procedures. It is an eye and skin irritant, and is toxic by inhalation and ingestion. In case of spills, ventilate area and mop up with wet mop.

**Glass Ionomer Cement:** Glass ionomer cement is a liquid/powder dental material. The liquid contains polycarboxylic acid, which may be an eye and skin irritant. Eye protection is recommended. In case of spills, mop up liquid with wet mop and sweep powder. Flush eyes with cold water if liquid or powder irritation occurs.

**Mercury:** Gloves should be worn whenever handling mercury. A source of contamination may be through inhalation of mercury vapors. If spill occurs, ventilate area and use a filter to remove mercury vapors from the air. Commercially available mercury spill kits are recommended for clean-up. **Do not use high-volume evacuation system.** Reassemble amalgam capsules after dispensing and store scrap amalgam under water in sealed container. Signs of excessive exposure to mercury include weakness, fatigue, loss of appetite, tremors of the fingers and eyelids, memory loss, depression, insomnia, dark pigmentation of the marginal gingiva, allergic manifestations, and convulsions.

**Nitrous Oxide:** A well ventilated area is required when working with nitrous oxide gas. Use of a scavenging system in the dental operatory is recommended to remove excess nitrous oxide gases exhaled by the patient. Store nitrous oxide tanks securely and away from heat or other flammable gases. Monitor equipment on a regular basis and check for leaks in hoses, masks, and tanks. NIOSH maximum exposure level of ambient gases is 25 parts per million.

**Polyether/Polysulfide Impression Material:** Gloves are recommended when working with methyl ethyl ketone impression materials. Adequate ventilation is also strongly recommended. If skin contact occurs, wash affected area with soap and water. Spills should be wiped up with a cloth or sponge and disposed of in a closed container.

**Radiographic Chemicals:** Hazardous chemicals such as acetic acid and hydroquinone are found in radiographic film processing fixer and developer solutions. Gloves and eye protection are recommended when working with these solutions. If eye contact occurs, flush eyes with cold water for fifteen minutes and seek medical attention. If skin contact occurs, remove contaminated clothing and wash affected area with soap and water. Spills should be covered with baking soda and cleaned up with absorbent materials which should later be disposed of in a closed container. Irritation to the nose and throat from vapors may also occur. Work in well-ventilated areas when handling radiographic chemicals.

**White Visible Light-Cured Materials:** Protective tinted eyewear is recommended when working with light-cured restorative materials. Potential damage to the retina of the eyes may occur. Avoid looking directly at the light during clinical application.

## Summary

- Properly discard chemicals which are no longer used or have expired.
- Use protective equipment to minimize chemical contact to skin and hands.
- Provide proper ventilation to minimize inhalation of chemicals and use respiratory protection and NIOSH-approved masks.
- If chemicals contact the eye, flush with cold water and seek medical attention as soon as possible.
- Neutralizing agents such as baking soda are effective for certain acid spills.
- A first-aid kit, portable oxygen resuscitation equipment, and fire extinguisher are essential in promoting general dental office safety.
- Use eye protection when working with acid etchants. If eye contact occurs, flush with cold water.
- Use a mask when working with alginate powders.
- Gloves and eye protection are recommended when working with disinfectants.
- When working with mercury, always wear gloves.
- A well-ventilated area is required when working with nitrous oxide gas.
- Hazardous chemicals such as acetic acid and hydroquinone are found in radiographis film processing fixer and developer solutions.
- Protective tinted eyewear is recommended when working with light-cured restorative materials.

# Review Questions

1. Define the key terms listed at the beginning of this chapter.

2. Explain why the bloodborne pathogen standard was initiated.

3. List the key requirements of OSHA's bloodborne pathogen standard.

4. Discuss how the dental health care worker can control occupational exposures to bloodborne pathogens by using personal protective equipment.

5. Give an example of an engineering control.

6. Describe the following work practice control requirements as they apply to a dental setting:

   • handwashing

   • flushing mucous membranes

   • prohibiting recapping, bending, shearing, or breaking of contaminated needles

   • placement of contaminated reusable sharps

   • prohibiting eating, drinking, smoking, applying cosmetics or handling contact lenses in areas where there is occupational exposure

   • prohibiting storage of food or drink in areas where infectious materials are present

   • storing, transporting, or shipping blood or other infectious materials

7. Explain why disinfectants are necessary for general housekeeping procedures in the dental environment.

8. What special precautions must be followed when disposing of contaminated sharps and other regulated waste?

9. If an occupational exposure incident occurs, where is the employer's incident report filed? How long must the employer keep these files?

10. How long must employee training records be kept by the employer?

11. Discuss why dental health care workers should be immunized with the Hepatitis B vaccine.

12. Describe the recommended method for handling contaminated laundry used as personal protective equipment in the dental setting. Your answer should include precautions for the employee handling the soiled laundry.

13. Identify key elements of an office written exposure control plan.

14. Give an example of an exposure incident.

15. What is the procedure for reporting an exposure incident to the employer by the employee? What specific responsibilities must the employer initiate?

16. Discuss key topics covered during an employee training session with respect to the bloodborne pathogen standard.

17. Explain why the hazard communication standard was initiated.

18. List the key requirements of OSHA's hazard communication standard.

19. Who is responsible for developing the material safety data sheets for each hazardous chemical?

20. What type of information is obtained from material safety data sheets?

21. Where should material safety data sheets be stored in the dental office?

22. Describe what is meant by reactivity data found on a material safety data sheet.

23. Why should dental health care workers read material safety data sheets?

24. List the main requirements of hazardous chemical labeling.

25. What guidelines must be followed in order to comply to OSHA's written hazard communication program?

26. List general office safety guidelines when handling hazardous chemicals in the dental office.

27. Identify essential equipment for promoting general dental office safety.

28. Identify and discuss the general product safety guidelines for the following:

    • acid etchants

    • acidulated fluoride

    • alginate impression material

    • BIS-GMA

    • bonding agents for porcelain

    • dental stone

    • disinfectants

    • formaldehyde

- glass ionomer cement

- mercury

- nitrous oxide

- polyether/polysulfide impression material

- radiographic chemicals

- white visible light-cured materials

# Dental Practice Management

10

## Key Terms ◀

| | | |
|---|---|---|
| *ACCOUNTS PAYABLE* | *EXCLUDED* | *NEGOTIATE* |
| *ACCOUNTS RECEIVABLE* | *FACSIMILE (FAX)* | *RECEIPT* |
| *CONFIDENTIALITY* | *INFORMED CONSENT* | *RECONCILE* |
| *CONSULTATION* | *INSURANCE CARRIER* | *REIMBURSE* |
| *CREDITS* | *INVENTORY* | *THIRD-PARTY PAYMENT* |
| *DEBIT* | *MALPRACTICE* | *VERIFICATION* |

## I. INTRODUCTION

Dentistry is a profession which functions with the qualities and atmosphere of a business. Dental practice management, as it is perceived in the world of modern dentistry, is crucial to establishing an efficient, effective practice. A dental practice cannot be effective unless it is efficient, and both can be accomplished only when the entire dental team uses basic operational business skills. Specialized roles have delegated advanced requirements and skills to perform efficiently as business assistant or dental office manager. Knowledge of accounting, recordkeeping, computer skills, third-party payment plans, patient communication skills, OSHA regulations, and related legal aspects of dentistry as they apply to these procedures is required of the business dental assistant. Appointment control, collections and financial payment arrangements, maintenance of the office inventory system, and implementing supervisory skills when indicated may be additional responsibilities. This chapter provides an overview of the business aspect of the professional dental practice and the role of the business office auxiliary.

## II.    THE OFFICE MANUAL

An office manual is a reference guide that contains detailed descriptions of all office policies and procedures. Information about the following aspects of the practice should be included.

1. The doctor's philosophy of practice (ie, goals and objectives).
2. Job descriptions for all members of the dental team.
3. Employment policies (eg, working hours, vacation, sick leave, overtime, holidays, dismissal, and termination).
4. Office policies for the staff (eg, dress code, conduct, staff meetings, continuing education).
5. Guidelines for appropriate office communication (eg, telephone technique, reception policies, written correspondence, patient education).
6. Policies for management of office records (eg, clinical and financial patient records, payment and collection procedures, accounts receivable, accounts payable, insurance coverage, recalls, inventory).
7. Guidelines for clinical procedures (eg, preparation of tray setups, sterilization techniques, prescriptions, laboratory interactions, OSHA regulations).
8. Medical emergency office protocol and procedures.
9. General office safety, fire safety, location of material safety data sheets (MSDS).
10. Quality assurance policies and procedures.

The guidelines set forth in the manual summarize office policies, reflect the characteristics of the practice, and enable the office to run smoothly from both a clinical and a management perspective. In addition, when a new employee joins the practice, the manual facilitates his or her integration into the practice. The office manual, which should be updated regularly, is an invaluable resource that promotes sound management and allows the office to run more efficiently.

The business assistant clearly performs an integral role in office administration. Tasks may vary as a function of the managerial style of the dentist, but the application of well-organized management techniques results in a successful office that provides fulfillment to the doctor, staff, and patients. It is the business assistant's responsibility to understand the principles of office administration and to employ them daily.

## III.    PERSONNEL MANAGEMENT

A written employment agreement is recommended for all new employees. The business office manager may be delegated the responsibility of reviewing portions of the employment agreement with the

---

### Office Manual Components

1. Office philosophy
2. Job descriptions
3. Employment policies
4. Office policies
5. Communication procedures
6. Maintenance office records
7. Clinical procedures
8. Medical emergency protocols
9. General office safety
10. Quality assurance

new employee. Employment agreements are signed by the employee and employer and are usually done in duplicate. One copy is to be given to the employee and the other copy is placed in the employee's permanent personnel file for the employer's records. The employment agreement includes an outline of the job duties, starting salary and range, working hours, probationary period, and information regarding termination procedures. It is important to note individual state dental practice acts for definitions of approved auxiliary duties under the general or direct supervision of a dentist.

If periodic employee evaluations are conducted in the office, they must be specified in the employment agreement. Some dental practices will provide an incentive or bonus plan and fringe benefits. Uniforms or reimbursement fees for certification renewal may be part of this plan. The employment agreement specifies this information to the employee. The employment agreement may also include state (EPA), or federal (OSHA) mandated regulatory agencies' specifications on certain work practice and engineering controls.

Personnel management practice requires that employers comply with federal regulatory agencies, which address fair employment and hiring practices. The Americans with Disabilities Act (ADA), which applies to fair hiring practices and elimination of discrimination against individuals who are disabled, must be recognized by the dental employer. Strict attention must be paid to federal laws regarding fair hiring and firing practices of all employees and appropriate steps should be taken to implement these practices into the dental office. Title II of the Americans with Disabilities Act mandates access to public service by the disabled.

## IV.  TELEPHONE COMMUNICATION

Every assistant should be aware that the telephone is an essential piece of equipment in the dental office. Without using it properly, a dentist cannot practice effectively. More than 95% of a dentist's business results from telephone calls, and the majority of new patients make the initial contact by telephone. It is therefore imperative that the telephone image conveyed by the auxiliary encourage a friendly, trusting attitude in the caller.

The production of dental services is the main function of the dentist. To maximize the delivery of services, it is necessary to keep delaying factors at a minimum level. Delaying factors include most telephone calls from patients, unexpected salespeople, family, and friends. All calls should be screened so that the doctor speaks only to patients who cannot be helped by the assistant.

When a caller questions fees, his or her concern should be addressed by an explanation that fees are contingent on procedures involved. Since a diagnosis cannot be determined over the telephone, a patient inquiring about fees should be scheduled for an examination and told that the dentist will discuss all fees before rendering any treatment.

If a telephone answering machine is used when the office is closed, the recorded message should be clear and understandable. The speaker should request pertinent information (eg, name, telephone number including the area code, and purpose of the call, or chief dental problem) and provide the caller with a clear understanding of what will happen as a result of the call (eg, the call will be returned, the caller should contact the doctor at another number, or the caller should contact another doctor who will see patients in emergency situations).

All phone conversations should be conducted in a professional, courteous manner. If a caller is to be placed on "hold," ask for the caller's permission first. If necessary, you may need to return a call and should ask the caller when it is best to return the call. When taking incoming office messages, it is best to log the following pertinent information: caller's name, date and time of message, action plan, and return phone number or follow-up recommendation to facilitate future contact with the caller.

If providing emergency instructions by phone for an avulsed tooth (a tooth which has been torn or knocked out of the socket by force), primary instructions should emphasize recommendations for: (1) a suitable transport media if unable to replant the avulsed tooth into the socket, and (2) the importance of professional emergency dental treatment. Suitable transport media includes: milk, saline, saliva (buccal vestibule) or Hank's Balanced Salt Solution. If the avulsed tooth can be replanted at the site of injury but is contaminated, rinse with water before replanting and seek professional emergency dental treatment.

A variety of options currently exist expanding telephone communication options. Office voice mail systems allow incoming calls to be directly forwarded to a specific staff member or set up to record messages from callers. **Facsimile (fax)** machines can be incorporated into a sophisticated office telephone system that allows written messages (paper communication) to be sent and received electronically.

## Summary

- Effective dental practice management incorporates a variety of business skills.
- An office manual summarizes office policies.
- The office manual facilitates training of new employees.
- A written employment agreement is recommended for all new employees.
- Employers must comply with federal employment and hiring laws.
- The Americans with Disabilities Act (ADA) applies to fair hiring practices and elimination of discrimination against individuals who are disabled.
- Approximately 95% of a dentists' business results from telephone calls.
- Recorded messages on answering machines should be clear and understandable.
- Phone conversations should be conducted in a professional and courteous manner.
- Voice mail systems allow incoming calls to be directed to a specific staff member.
- Fax machines allow written communication to be sent and received electronically.
- An avulsed tooth injury requires professional emergency dental treatment.

■ Suitable transport media for an avulsed tooth includes milk, saline, saliva (buccal vestibule), or Hank's Balanced salt solution.

## V.  PATIENT RECEPTION

The business assistant is the key public relations member of the office team because he or she makes the first contact with patients, both on the telephone and in the reception area. During the initial interaction with new patients, first impressions are very important, and consequently the assistant should make an effort to be courteous and pleasant at all times. The first meeting is a time for exchanging information and familiarizing the patient with office procedures. A warm friendly greeting by auxiliaries can engender the same feelings toward the doctor even before the patient and doctor meet. Apprehensive patients are extended a feeling of reassurance and calmness by the office assistant.

Important patient data such as medical dental histories are often taken at the front desk reception area. Patient confidentiality should always be observed and respected. The front desk reception area may also allow for communication regarding financial management of individual patient accounts and insurance coverage information. Dental pre- and post-treatment patient instructions are addressed by the office assistant and may include specific patient education information relative to their dental visit.

The reception area must be clean, and patients should be greeted promptly on arrival. Patient arrivals should be made known to the doctor as quickly as possible via a signal system. If the dentist is delayed, patients who are waiting should be notified and told approximately how long it will be before they will be seen by the doctor. This information will clarify to all patients that the office has respect for both their time and the doctor's, and this consideration is always appreciated.

## VI.  PATIENT RECORDS

A series of records should be maintained for each patient. A case history form that includes the patient's past and present medical and dental health histories should be updated periodically to avoid potential medical emergencies and legal problems. **Informed consent** ◀ implies that the patient has had a thorough explanation of the required treatment, risks, and expectations if the proposed treatment is not done. When the patient has been informed of the course of treatment needed, it is necessary to obtain the patient's consent to treatment in writing, provided the patient is of legal age.

Diagnostic materials include x-ray films, information noted at the clinical examination, and study models. A patient information sheet contains the record of existing conditions and a prioritized treatment plan designed for each patient on the basis of the doctor's diagnosis. The plan enables the dentist to systematically meet the dental needs of the patient and enables the business assistant to facilitate the course of treatment by knowing the procedures required, the order of procedures, the person who will perform each procedure (ie, the dentist, an assistant, or a hygienist), the time required for each procedure, and the total fee for services to be rendered.

Permanent record cards are maintained for each patient and contain specific notations of all treatment performed, the date on which it was performed, materials used, the prognosis, and other relevant information. Entries regarding emergency treatment or the patient's refusal to consent to recommended treatment should also be noted.

Individually and collectively, these records protect both the patient and the dentist should treatment discrepancies arise. Patient records are confidential histories of financial and treatment experiences that cannot be released or made public without the patient's permission. Before any records leave the office (eg, for insurance purposes or consultation with a specialist), duplicate copies should ► be made for legal protection. A **consultation** is often sought between two or more health care professionals for specific advice regarding a patient's proposed treatment and diagnosis. Keep in mind that the dental record is permissible as evidence in a court of law ► and is usually the single most valuable piece of evidence in a **malpractice** case. All entries must be made in ink. If an entry is corrected, the initials of the party making the change must be recorded.

If dental records are computerized, consideration towards ade- ► quate security and **confidentiality** of the dental records should be given. Appropriate measures may include issuance of individual passwords to allow a limited number of personnel to access dental record information. Passwords prohibit unauthorized users from accessing confidential or important information from the computer.

## VII.  RECORD AND BOOKKEEPING SYSTEMS

A record and bookkeeping system encompasses all paperwork pertaining to the dental practice, ranging from the appointment book, which is usually the first place that the patient's name appears, to collection control, which is often the last. The system must be completely standardized and organized, since accurate and adequate records provide a comprehensive history of past and present patient treatment, production records that enable the dentist to assess expenses periodically through cost accounting, and precise tax information. These records also can prevent or resolve malpractice involvement. All records must be complete and accurately documented in ink for legal purposes.

Basic filing systems should be kept as simple as possible. Alphabetical or numerical coding systems may also be initiated. File guides depicting the patient's name or identification code must be clearly visible. Active and inactive patient record files should be maintained. Permanent patient records should never be destroyed, even if deemed inactive.

Office records must be protected against loss and especially against fire. Fireproof file cabinets with locks are recommended. Every office should have a security alarm system to protect against theft.

## VIII.   APPOINTMENT BOOK AND DAY SHEET

The appointment book is the control center of office activity. A mismanaged appointment book can destroy a potentially fine practice by wasting the doctor's productive time or by creating a schedule that results in a waiting room filled with unhappy patients. For optimum control, the appointment book should be the responsibility of the business assistant, who has an overview of all doctor–patient activity, knowledge of patient availability in relation to office availability, and an understanding of the amount of time necessary for treatment planned.

Time and motion studies have shown that one of the most efficient formats of an appointment book is the week-at-a-glance style. The format enables the assistant to balance the workload appropriately by noting available time during the week. The patient's name, phone number, and procedure scheduled for that time slot should be printed in pencil to provide easy reading and to allow any changes to be entered neatly. Appointments which have been confirmed should also be identified.

In advance, certain periods of time should be matrixed or blocked out (eg, lunch and dinner hours, holidays, when the office will be closed, vacation time, and professional meetings when the doctor will not be in the office). Time should be prioritized to reflect the periods of the day that are valued most highly and the type of patients who will be appointed during those times. The preferences of the doctor and working schedules of business people should be reflected in this determination.

Elderly patients and young children should be scheduled early in the day, a time when they will be most cooperative. Patients with special needs, such as medical problems or physical impairments, also should be considered when scheduling dental appointments. In addition, a philosophy for emergency patients should be developed. Some offices reserve buffer periods for unexpected emergencies, whereas others work them into existing schedules.

Broken appointments and cancellations may disrupt the most organized office. Patients who repeatedly break appointments or cancel them with insufficient notice should be made aware that this is unacceptable behavior. Time created, however, should be used efficiently, and a call list that contains patients' names, telephone numbers, and times they are available on short notice should be created for maximum use of office resources.

Most efficient offices schedule patients in time units. The most frequent time units selected include a period of 10 or 15 minutes. A patient being appointed for a procedure requiring 45 minutes should be scheduled for three units of time in the appointment book if the office is on a 15-minute unit increment of time schedule. On a 10-minute unit of time increment schedule, a 40-minute appointment would require 4 units. Unit scheduling provides a realistic mechanism for controlling the workload and allows the dental team to adhere to the schedule throughout the day. Scheduling a patient for a 15-minute appointment when the actual time needed is 30 minutes is one of the reasons that some offices consistently work overtime. To alleviate improper scheduling and ensure that each patient will be appointed appropriately for the next visit, the doctor or chairside assistant must provide the person controlling the appointment book with information about the procedure planned in units of time required for the patient's next appointment.

If indicated, adequate time should be allotted between appointments to complete necessary dental laboratory work for the scheduled dental patients of the day. The dental auxiliary should verify that the laboratory casework that is being done by a commercial dental laboratory outside of the office is returned to the office by the time the patient is appointed.

The day sheet is a replica of the appointment book for the day and should be placed in each treatment room. This schedule provides the dentist and auxiliaries in the operatories with the information necessary to eliminate checking the appointment book to determine who is expected, the time of the appointment, and the treatment planned. The day sheet also enables the staff to plan ahead and minimize delaying factors by preparing the necessary instruments and materials for the next scheduled patient in advance.

## IX. THE RECALL SYSTEM

A responsive recall system is essential to every dental office. It reflects a supportive attitude that encourages patients to maintain proper oral health for a lifetime. At the end of each series of treatments, the dentist or the assistant should remind the patient that they should return for an examination after a given interval of time. The atmosphere created should be motivating and reflect concern for the patient's health, but it should be clear that maintenance and recall are a dual responsibility, and patients who fail to respond may compromise their oral health.

Recall methods vary. Some offices telephone patients, others send written reminders, and others use a combination of telephone and mail notices. Once the method of recall is chosen, a recall file that can be used and updated easily should be established. A patient's recall card should be separate from his or her clinical chart, and each family member should have an individual recall card, since the length of time between examinations may vary.

A standard recall method of record keeping includes the two-card system for each patient: one card is designated by the month during which the recall visit should occur, and the other is alphabetical by patient name. For reference, the monthly card should be filed in a box divided in the same manner. Each card should include the patient's name, complete home and business address, telephone number, and preferred type of reminder (written or phone). The recall card can also be used to keep a record of the patient's recall pattern.

Alphabetical cards can be filed in a revolving desk file and should include the patient's name, type of reminder preferred, and date of the last appointment. This file also serves as a tickler file and is easily accessible if a patient should call to inquire about the recall or to request treatment earlier than the scheduled time. Some newer record-keeping systems employ the computer to update monthly patient recalls and send out reminders for the patients who have not made an appointment. Computerized recall systems may also be maintained and used for filing patient recall data and mailing recall reminders.

## Summary

- Patient confidentiality should always be observed and respected.
- The dental receptionist gathers important patient information such as medical and dental history, insurance coverage, purpose of the dental visit and/or chief complaint.
- Informed consent implies that the patient has had a thorough explanation of the required treatment and risks.
- Diagnostic materials include x-rays and study models.
- Patient treatment plans must be prioritized and include a record of the total fees for services rendered.
- Patient dental records contain confidential information.
- Before dental records leave the dental office, duplicate copies should be made for legal protection.
- Dental record entries must be legible and made in ink.
- All office records should be protected against fire and theft.
- Filing systems may be alphabetical or numerical.
- Never destroy a dental record.
- Dental record files should be separated into "active" and "inactive" filing systems.
- The appointment book is the responsibility of the business assistant.
- Elderly patients and young children should be scheduled early in the day when they are more cooperative.
- Schedule patients with special needs accordingly.
- Matrix the appointment book if buffer time is needed.
- Establish an office policy for broken appointments and cancellations.
- Patients' treatment may be scheduled in an appointment book using time unit intervals of 10 or 15 minutes.
- Verify that all dental laboratory casework has been returned to the office by the time of the patient's next appointment.
- At the end of each series of appointments, remind the patient that they should return for an examination after a given interval of time-recall appointment.
- A patient's recall card should be separate from their clinical chart.
- Each family member should have an individual recall card.
- The office recall system may be computerized.

## X.  ACCOUNTS RECEIVABLE AND ACCOUNTS PAYABLE MANAGEMENT

Accurate financial records must be maintained for both efficiency and legal protection, and the actual bookkeeping is only as valuable as the detail and accuracy with which it is maintained. The simplest system is single-entry bookkeeping, which records only payments. The double-entry system records both the debit (charges) and credit (payments) for each office transaction. The two entries provide the necessary information to balance the financial records and provide duplicate records in the event that a patient's card is lost or destroyed.

Many offices use a pegboard system, a form of double entry that allows two or more office records to be written at one time through the use of carbon paper and pegs that stabilize punched forms in the correct position. Some large dental practices use electronic data-processing systems involving computers to record production and financial data, recall dates, and patient account histories.

▶ A daily **accounts receivable** bookkeeping system includes the following basic entry information: patient name, treatment charges, payment, and adjustments to the account. Pre-printed bookkeeping systems also incorporate either charge slips, encounter forms, or posting slips, which are used to transmit information from the treatment area to the front office. These forms are printed in duplicate, and one copy remains in the office for posting and the second copy

▶ provides the patient with a **receipt** (written account of amount paid) of the financial transactions for the day and subsequent account record.

Every office has a policy about payments. A dental practice cannot survive if there is an inordinate amount of accounts receivable (money owed to the dentist for treatment completed). Fees charged for services rendered represent the dentist's earnings, but only payments actually received constitute income. For the practice to be profitable, income must exceed expenses (overhead), which is the cost of the resources needed to produce dentistry, including rent, salaries, supplies, laboratory procedures, and so forth. The expenses

▶ (overhead) of a dental practice constitute the **accounts payable.**

Credit experts indicate that delinquent accounts over 90 days old are difficult and often impossible to collect. In order to minimize accounts receivable, all patients should be informed of the exact financial obligation before treatment is begun. The business assistant

▶ has the responsibility to **negotiate** (discuss and conclude a business transaction) with the patient regarding the preferred method of payment. Various payment policies and methods should be offered as a means of making the responsibility less burdensome. Payment methods include cash, checks, money orders, credit cards, and bank plans. There are many payment policies, but those shown in Table 10–1 are the most common.

Although proper payment arrangements may be made, some patients fail to fulfill their obligations of honoring the method of payment to which they have agreed. The business assistant should monitor payment arrangements continuously. As a patient makes the next appointment, the assistant should check to see whether payment is due. If the patient is defaulting and payment is not forthcoming, the assistant should address the issue. Patients should not be given the option of whether to pay but rather of how to pay. If patients offer excuses rather than payments, they should be informed that they may either mail the payment (a stamped, self-addressed envelope should be provided) or bring it in at the next visit.

If a patient continues to default, the assistant should remind the patient that arrangements were agreed upon and determine whether there is a need to renegotiate the contract and ask the patient to select an alternate method of payment. Although many people tend to pay dental obligations last, most will adhere as agreed after being reminded of their responsibilities.

Statements should be used minimally as a mechanism for reminding patients of balance to date, when a patient has stopped treatment before completion, or when they have finished treatment sooner than expected. Statements are used to remind patients of di-

TABLE 10–1. PAYMENT POLICY METHODS

| METHOD | DEFINITION |
|---|---|
| Advanced payment | Payment before treatment is the most desirable, since billing, collection problems and accounts receivable are eliminated. |
| Fixed amount | The total fee is divided by the approximate number of sessions projected for completion of the treatment, and a fixed amount is expected from the patient at each visit, regardless of the actual charge for particular treatment rendered during the visit. |
| Divided payment | The total fee is divided into three amounts. The initial payment, usually larger than the other two, is collected when treatment commences. The balance, which is divided in half, is due when treatment is half completed and a visit or two before treatment is completed. |
| Open account | Patients are sent statements (forms indicating the financial status of their accounts) after treatment is rendered. This method often results in high accounts receivable, since most patients are unaware of their obligations until they receive statements, are often unprepared to pay for services rendered, or take a substantial amount of time to complete payment. |

vided payment agreements, noting the dates and amounts of expected payments.

A small percentage of patients complete treatment with an outstanding balance. These patients should be sent several statements at regular intervals (eg, every 30 days). If the patient does not respond, telephone follow-up should be initiated. If these efforts are unsuccessful, the patient should be informed that if payment is not received on a specified date, the matter will be referred for collection. Most people are concerned with collection referral, since their credit rating can be jeopardized.

Computerized management systems may also be employed for billing purposes and efficient processing of insurance forms. Posting of payments directly into the doctor's bank account may also be accomplished via the computer. Security issues must be considered when using computers in the dental office. Back-up files should be created whenever possible to ensure that important information and files are not lost. Internal audits should be periodically monitored.

If bank deposits are not being made via a computerized system, it is necessary to complete a bank deposit slip. The bank deposit slip posts an itemized list of all collected currency and received payment checks. The date and total amount of the deposit is clearly entered on the pre-printed office deposit slip. A duplicate copy of the completed deposit slip is kept for future reference. Deposits are done on a daily basis.

Each office may establish an office policy regarding a change fund. A change fund is the specified amount of cash used on a daily basis in the office for transactions involving change. The change fund is not recorded on the bank deposit slip.

If the office uses a petty cash fund for small expenses, a petty cash voucher and receipt for the items purchased must be maintained. The petty cash voucher must include the date, amount spent, who spent the petty cash, and what the item was used for. A petty cash fund may be used to pay for small items such as office-requested C.O.D. deliveries or postage.

▶     To **reconcile** (balance) a bank statement, check the number of
▶ each outstanding check and enter all debits on to the register. **Verification** (to check for accuracy) of all deposits made should also be
▶ reviewed. **Debits** are considered items which have been deducted from the account. These items may include the bank service charges.
▶ **Credits** are considered items which have been deposited into the account. Credits to the account may also include earned interest. It is best to reconcile (balance) the bank statement with the checkbook as soon as the statement is received. Outstanding and cancelled checks must be considered when balancing the bank statement.

Accurate records must be maintained according to federal regulations relative to employee's earned pay and payroll taxes. The business assistant may be responsible for preparing the payroll and maintaining the employee's record of hours worked, earnings, and deductions. A private accountant is often used for summarizing monthly and annual financial reports for the dental practice. Each employee is required to complete an employee's withholding (W-4 form). The form is a federal requirement and allows the employer to legally deduct a portion of the employee's estimated withholding tax.

## Insurance Deductibles

An amount of eligible expenses that must be paid by the patient before the insurance plan will pay benefits

## Insurance Co-payment

An amount paid by a health plan member for services. May be a fixed, flat fee.

# XI.   THIRD PARTY CARRIERS

An increased number of people have dental insurance coverage, and
▶ it is estimated that this population will be enlarged annually. The **insurance carrier** (insurance company that offers dental plans) is chosen by the employer for their employees. The insurance carrier agrees to cover and pay for benefits claimed under the plan. As a result, insurance claim management is an important duty of the business assistant. Managing insurance coverage in a positive manner often results in practice growth because:

1. Patients accept comprehensive care, since the cost of treatment is defrayed by coverage
2. People who previously did not seek oral health care are taking advantage of third party coverage
3. Accounts receivable are often reduced substantially due to payments received directly from insurance carriers.

Many forms of insurance coverage exist. Insurance companies
▶ may **reimburse** (repay) the doctor or the patient for dental services rendered. The amount of reimbursement may be based on usual, customary, or reasonable fees (UCR), which is an amount considered standard for the procedure in a given community or a fixed amount determined by the carrier for each procedure.

The insured patient (subscriber) should be made aware of the dental insurance policy individual benefits and limitations. Individual policy deductibles and co-payments must also be understood by the dental patient at the time of financial arrangements regarding the proposed treatment plan being made. Certain dental procedures and services may be **excluded** and indicate that the carrier **will not** pay ◀ for this type of dental treatment. Many insurance carriers also maintain a maximum. The maximum amount limits the dollar amount of payment on dental services and may be set on an annual maximum scale limiting payment of treatment even for covered dental services under the insurance plan.

The business assistant should be familiar with the organization of different types of coverage and understand how they affect the payments between the dentist and the patient. Dental patients may also maintain "dual coverage" benefits, indicating that the patient has dental insurance coverage under more than one plan. It is important to differentiate which insurance carrier is the primary carrier and which insurance carrier is considered the secondary carrier. For children with dual coverage, the "birthday rule" is used to determine which insurance carrier should be considered primary. The birthday rule designates that the insurance carrier for the parent who has a birthday earlier in the year is to be considered the primary carrier for the child.

Most insurance carriers use specific procedure codes established by the American Dental Association (ADA). The Code on Dental Procedures and Nomenclature is published in the Current Dental Terminology (CDT, 2nd edition) guidebook.

For maximum efficiency, a patient's insurance forms should not be located with the clinical records. A separate insurance file should be maintained and checked periodically to ensure prompt claim processing. Insurance claims are a form of accounts receivable—money owed to the dental practice. For this reason, insurance claims should be processed as quickly as possible. EDI-electronic data interchange may be used to process insurance claims the same day the patient receives treatment.

The insured patient should be aware of individual benefits, and the business assistant can often increase or clarify this understanding. This knowledge encourages acceptance of total treatment plans because the patient understands his or her financial responsibilities and those of the insurer. The doctor's treatment planning may also be affected by this type of coverage. When a patient calls for an appointment, he or she should be told that all forms, benefit booklets, and other relevant information should be brought to the office on the first visit. The business assistant then has the opportunity to initiate the payment process and alleviate or diminish any potential problems.

There are several different kinds of **third-party payment** plans. ◀ Some plans are organized on a prepayment basis, such as an HMO (Health Maintenance Organization) or PPO (Preferred Provider Organization) where the doctor receives a fixed amount of money for each patient for a specified period of time. An IPA (Independent Practice Association) is an HMO that contracts with provider groups to see HMO patients in addition to private practice patients. Under the IPA model, groups of dentists provide dental services collectively on a capitation basis to a selected enrolled population group.

A DMO or DHMO (Dental Health Maintenance Organization) is a prepaid dental plan run on an HMO model. Under capitation programs, the dentist has contracted to provide dental services to subscribers in payment on a per capita basis. With capitation, the dentist receives the same amount of money regardless of the type and

---

## Third Party Payment Plans

HMO—Health Maintenance Organization
PPO—Preferred Provider Organization
IPA—Independent Practice Association
DHMO—Dental Health Maintenance Organization
DRP—Direct Reimbursement Plan

amount of care delivered. Patients covered by this type of insurance seek care only from participating dentists who constitute a closed panel.

Direct reimbursement plans involve no specific type of insurance plan. This benefit agreement is between the employer and the employee. When the patient completes dental treatment, a payment is made to the dentist by the patient. The employer, in turn, will reimburse the employee for the specified dollar amount benefit according to company policy.

## XII. INVENTORY SYSTEMS

For efficiency, every office must maintain a well-organized **inventory** system. An inventory system can be created simply by using index cards or the pages of a loose leaf binder. Each major disposable item used in the office has its own card or page and contains the following information:

1. The name of the item (eg, anesthetic)
2. The brand name (eg, Carbocaine 2%)
3. The name of the supplier and the supplier's address and telephone number
4. How the item is sold (eg, box, case, package)
5. The quantity to order for the most advantageous price
6. The time at which the item should be reordered (the reorder point) (eg, when only three cases of a material are left)
7. Back orders, which are items previously ordered but not shipped by the supplier because of temporary unavailability

When an item is removed from the supply storage area, it should be recorded in the supply log book in order to keep accurate records of current stock on hand. When new supplies are ordered, the assistant must not change the inventory record until the items are actually delivered in order to keep an accurate accounting of what is on hand and what is back ordered.

Careful planning and periodic evaluation of the office inventory system can result in several advantages for the dental practice. For example, information about the quantity of any given material used in a time period enables the office to take advantage of savings resulting from quantity buying. Awareness of the rise of the price of dental materials enables the dentist to adjust fees using cost accounting methods. An efficient office supply system allows the practice to run smoothly by preventing critical shortages of necessary supplies during patient treatment procedures.

In order to maintain an efficient office supply system, a perpetual inventory should be performed at regular intervals. If at all possible, stocking space should be marked with the proper item name or item number to correspond with the inventory control card. This will assist in accountability of the inventory and ensure control. In addition, storage space should be considered when ordering new supplies and dental materials. Factors such as storage location are critical to certain dental materials and supplies. X-ray film, for example, should not be stored in an area which is subject to scatter radiation,

### Inventory Identification System

1. Name of item
2. Brand name
3. Name of supplier
4. How item is sold (eg, case)
5. Quantity to order
6. Reorder point
7. Back order log

heat, or excessive light. Appropriate security measures (eg, locked cabinet) and strict inventory control should be conducted for prescription drugs stored in the office.

To assist you in preparing for the Specialty Examination in Dental Practice Management, it is recommended that you review Chapter 3, Infection Control; Chapter 5, Chairside Assisting; Chapter 6, Dental Radiology; Chapter 8, Medical Emergencies; and Chapter 9, Occupational Safety.

## Summary

- A single-entry bookkeeping system records only payments.
- A double-entry bookkeeping system records both the debit (charges) and credit (payments).
- Computerized bookkeeping systems are used for maintaining patient account histories and billing.
- Posting slips are used to record the patient's financial transactions.
- Money owed to the dentist for treatment is referred to as accounts receivable.
- For a practice to be profitable, income must exceed overhead.
- Financial arrangements regarding method of payment should be finalized prior to beginning treatment.
- Statements are used to remind patients of divided payment agreements.
- Security issues must be considered when using computers in the dental office.
- The bank deposit slip posts an itemized list of all collected currency and received payment checks.
- A change fund is used in-office to provide transactions involving change.
- To reconcile a bank statement, check the number of all outstanding checks, enter all debits on to the register, and verify deposits.
- Debits are items which have been deducted from the account.
- Credits are items which have been deposited into the account.
- A petty cash fund is used for small office expenses.
- Payroll taxes must be deducted according to federal regulations.
- Reimbursement may be based on (UCR) usual, customary, or reasonable fees.
- The "birthday rule" is used to determine which insurance carrier is the primary carrier for a child under dual coverage benefits.
- The (CDT) Current Dental Terminology Guidebook is published by the ADA and contains insurance codes.
- Insurance claims are a form of accounts receivable and should be processed quickly.
- Pre-payment plans include HMOs or PPOs.
- Capitation exists under the IPA model.
- Direct reimbursement plans do not involve an insurance carrier.
- An inventory system is required for ordering dental supplies.
- Identify low inventory stock with a reorder point.
- Do not store x-ray film near excessive light or heat.
- Prescription drugs, if stored in the office, must be in a locked cabinet.

# Review Questions

1. Discuss the importance of incorporating business skills into the dental practice.

2. Describe the role of the dental office manager and/or business assistant.

3. What is the purpose of an office manual?

4. List several key components of the office manual.

5. Why is an employment agreement recommended?

6. What does an employment agreement between the employer and employee include?

7. Discuss the importance of complying with state or federal mandated regulatory agencies (eg, OSHA).

8. Describe how the Americans with Disabilities Act applies to the hiring and management of personnel.

9. How should the office telephone communications be handled?

10. What is meant by office voice mail?

11. What is a facsimile (fax)?

12. Describe the emergency instructions for an avulsed tooth.

13. How should patients be greeted in the office reception area?

14. Why must patient confidentiality always be observed and respected?

15. How should the business assistant handle the nervous or apprehensive patient?

16. Define the term "informed consent."

17. Identify items included as part of the patient's permanent dental record.

18. What is the legal importance of the patient dental record?

19. Why must dental records be duplicated before they leave the office?

20. What security measures must be incorporated if the patient dental record is computerized?

21. Describe basic filing systems for dental records.

22. What special precautions should be taken to protect records against hazards such as fire?

23. Discuss the importance of appointment control in the dental office.

24. Why is it necessary to matrix blocks of time in a schedule?

25. Describe the basic appointment book entries for each patient scheduled.

26. What is a day sheet? How does the day sheet assist the chairside auxiliary?

27. When should very young patients or elderly patients be scheduled?

28. Identify scheduling methods for the patient who has a dental emergency.

29. How can broken appointments or cancellations be managed?

30. How do units of time (increments) assist in scheduling specific dental procedures?

31. Why is it important to check with the dental laboratory prior to scheduling the patient?

32. Describe the function of a recall system.

33. What is meant by a single-entry bookkeeping system and a double-entry bookkeeping system?

34. Define the term accounts receivable.

35. What is considered a delinquent account? How can this type of account be avoided?

36. Why are dental statements used?

37. What steps can be taken to protect the data within the computer system if used for billing and insurance claims?

38. List the basic steps for preparing a daily bank deposit.

39. What is the purpose of a change fund?

40. How is the petty cash fund managed?

41. How do you reconcile a bank statement?

42. What guidelines must be followed when preparing the payroll?

43. Describe different methods of third-party payments:

    - HMO-

    - DMO-

    - IPA-

- PPO-

- Direct Reimbursement Plan-

- Capitation-

44. What is meant by the term "UCR"?

45. Define the following terms as they apply to a dental insurance policy:

- benefits-

- limitations-

- deductibles-

- co-payments-

- excluded-

- maximum-

- dual coverage-

- primary carrier-

- secondary carrier-

- "birthday rule"-

46. What is the ADA Code on Dental Procedures and Nomenclature used for?

47. Why is it important for a dental office to establish and maintain an inventory system?

48. Define the reorder point.

49. Where is the best place to store the x-ray film?

50. When storing controlled substances in the dental office what security measures must be followed?

# Glossary

Glossary will assist test candidates' understanding of content material found in Chapter 4, Infection Control, and Chapter 9, Occupational Safety.

**ADA:** American Dental Association

**Aerobe:** microorganism that can live and grow only where free oxygen is present

**Aerosol:** particles of microscopic size dispensed in solution or suspended in air. Dental aerosol is generated during use of dental armamentarium, for example, handpieces, sonics, air/water syringe

**AIDS:** Acquired Immunodeficiency Syndrome. The final stage of disease from the Human Immunodeficiency Virus.

**Allergy:** hypersensitivity to a specific substance, for example, latex

**Antibody:** specialized protein produced in response to an antigen, creating an immunity

**Antigen:** substance that induces the formation of an immune response

**Antimicrobial:** capable of suppressing the growth of microorganisms

**Antiseptic:** compounds that inhibit the growth of bacteria

**Asepsis:** the absence of infection or pathogenic microorganisms

**Aseptic:** absence of pathogens

**Asymptomatic:** no symptoms of infection

**Autoclave:** an instrument for sterilization using moist heat under pressure

**AZT:** ZDV-Zibovudine approved drug for initial therapy of primary HIV-1 infection

**Bacteremia:** presence of bacteria in the bloodstream

**Bactericidal:** a substance that destroys bacteria

**Bacteriostatic:** agent that stops the growth of bacteria

**Barrier protection:** protection against contamination provided by personal protective equipment

**Bioburden:** microbial or organic material on an object prior to decontamination

**Biohazard:** contaminated substance that poses a biologic risk and potential for disease transmission

**Biological Indicator:**   monitoring device for heat and gas sterilizers, for example, vial containing endospores

**Booster Vaccination:**   vaccine injected at appropriate intervals after the primary immunization to sustain an immune response

**Candidiasis:**   oral lesion associated with AIDS caused by the Candida species of yeastlike fungi

**CDC:**   Centers for Disease Control and Prevention (CDCP)

**Chemical Indicator:**   monitoring device for the process of checking temperature range during use of sterilizers, for example, autoclave striped tape, color change stripe on autoclave bags.

**Communicable:**   infectious, capable of being spread or transmitted

**Contamination:**   introduction of blood or infectious agent on an item or surface

**Cross Contamination:**   spread of disease through contact with contaminated items or surfaces

**Decontamination:**   use of physical or chemical means to destroy pathogens; removal of bioburden from surfaces

**DHCW:**   Dental Health Care Worker

**Disinfectant:**   chemical agent applied to inanimate objects for the destruction of microorganisms. Disinfectants do not destroy bacterial spores.

**Disinfection:**   the destruction or removal of pathogenic organisms by a chemical substance

**Droplet Infection:**   disease transmission through small liquid droplets, as from sneezing and coughing

**ELISA:**   Enzyme-Linked Immunosorbent Assay, detection test for the presence of HIV antibody

**Engineering Controls:**   controls that isolate or remove the hazard from the workplace, for example, sharps disposal container

**EPA:**   Environmental Protection Agency

**Epidemic:**   rapid spreading of a disease among a population

**Exposure Control Plan:**   a written plan required by OSHA that describes how exposure to bloodborne disease agents will be controlled at the workplace

**Exposure Incident:**   contact with infectious agent or blood during the performance of duties

**FDA:**   Food and Drug Administration

**Fungicidal:**   capable of killing fungi

**Hairy Leukoplakia:**   oral lesion associated with HIV positive infection, white in color, commonly found on lateral borders of tongue

**Hazard Communication Standard:**   OSHA law directing employers to provide employees with information on chemical hazards in the workplace

**Hazardous Waste:**   contaminated waste which poses a biologic risk to the environment

**HBIG:**   Hepatitis B Immune Globulin, prepared from plasma known to contain a high titer of antibody against HBSAg

**HBV:**   Hepatitis B Virus

| **HCW:** | Health Care Worker |
|---|---|
| **HIV:** | Human Immunodeficiency Virus |
| **HIV+:** | Seropositive indicates a positive test for the HIV antibody |
| **Host:** | the organic body upon which or in which parasites live |
| **Immunity:** | having antibodies to protect against a disease |
| **Immuno-deficiency:** | inability of immune system to respond to an antigen |
| **Incubation Stage:** | time between an infectious exposure and the appearance of signs and symptoms of disease |
| **Infection:** | condition in which the body is invaded by a pathogen |
| **Infection Control:** | to control disease by performing specific procedures and eliminating the spread of contaminated agents |
| **Infectious Waste:** | regulated waste contaminated with blood, saliva, or other infectious agents |
| **Kaposi's Sarcoma:** | oral lesion associated with HIV infection, malignant and of blood vessel origin |
| **Microbial Growth:** | cell division resulting in an increase in the number of cells |
| **MMWR:** | Morbidity and Mortality Weekly Report published weekly by CDC |
| **MSDS:** | Material Safety Data Sheets which indicate chemical properties and hazards |
| **NIOSH:** | National Institute for Occupational Safety and Health |
| **Occupational Exposure:** | reasonably anticipated skin, eye, mucous membrane, or parenteral contact with blood or other infectious materials that may result from the performance of an employee's duties |
| **OPIM:** | other potentially infectious materials |
| **OSHA:** | Occupational Safety and Health Administration |
| **Parenteral:** | exposure as the result of breaking or piercing the skin barrier through events such as needlesticks, human bites, cuts, and abrasions |
| **Pathogen:** | microorganism that is capable of causing a disease |
| **Pathologic Waste:** | includes extracted teeth, biopsy specimens |
| **PPE:** | Personal Protective Equipment, or specialized clothing or equipment worn by an employee for protection against a hazard, for example, gloves, mask, eyewear, uniforms, gowns, resuscitation bags, ventilation devices, face shields |
| **Post-Exposure Evaluation:** | follow-up report after an exposure incident given to the employee by the employer |
| **Regulated Waste:** | contaminated hazardous waste which requires OSHA disposal methods; includes liquid or semi-liquid blood or other potentially infectious materials |
| **Sepsis:** | presence of infectious disease-producing microorganisms |
| **Sharps:** | objects capable of penetrating the skin, for example, needles, broken glass |
| **Sharps Container:** | puncture-resistant container for the disposal of needles, scalpel blades, ortho wires, or other sharp items |

**Shelf Life:**         storage time period of a product before activation or use which denotes that it will still retain effectiveness

**Source Individual:**  any individual, living or dead, whose blood or other potentially infectious materials may be a source of occupational exposure to the employee

**Sporicide:**          agent capable of killing spores

**Sterilant:**          an agent capable of killing all microorganisms

**Sterilization:**      the removal or destruction of all microorganisms

**Surface Asepsis:**    procedures that prevent the spread of infectious agents on environmental surfaces

**Toxic:**              pertaining to a poison or toxin

**Toxic Waste:**        waste which is poisonous or toxic

**Transmission:**       a transfer from one individual to another

**Tuberculocidal:**     agent that can kill *Mycobacterium tuberculosis*

**Universal Precautions:**  consideration of all patients as being infected with pathogens; therefore applying infection control procedures to all patients

**Use Life:**           time period a solution is effective after activation or preparation

**Vaccine:**            substance that contains an antigen to which the immune system can respond

**Vaccination:**        the production of immunity to a specific disease by placing a vaccine into the body

**Virucidal:**          agent that kills viruses

**Virus:**              submicroscopic organism which causes infectious diseases

**Zibovudine:**         AZT/ZDV approved drug for initial therapy of primary HIV-1 infection

# Bibliography

American Dental Assistants Association Department of Continuing Education, *ICE PACK,* 1995.

American Heart Association. *A Student Handbook for Cardiopulmonary Resuscitation and First Aid for Choking,* 1993.

American National Red Cross. *American Red Cross Standard First Aid Workbook.* 1988.

American Red Cross. *Advanced First Aid and Emergency Care,* 2nd ed. New York: Doubleday and Co, Inc, 1980.

Anthony CP, Thibodeau GA. *Structure and Function of the Body,* 6th ed. St. Louis: CV Mosby Co, 1980.

Atchison KA. *Radiographic Safety.* Western Dental Education Center Correspondence Course. Los Angeles: Department of Veteran Affairs, West Los Angeles VA Medical Center, 1987.

Boucher CO. *Boucher's Clinical Dental Terminology: Glossary of Accepted Terms in All Disciplines of Dentistry,* 4th ed. C.V. Mosby, St. Louis, 1993.

Brown SK. *Infection Control in Dental Practices,* 1993 Health Studies Institute, Inc. Miami, Florida.

Butsumyo D, Deboom G, Lynne S, Parrot K. *Principles and Practice of Dental Radiography.* Los Angeles: Western Dental Education Center Correspondence Course. Department of Veteran Affairs, West Los Angeles VA Medical Center, 1988.

Caplan CM. *Dental Practice Management Encyclopedia,* Penn Well, 1985.

Carter LM, Yaman P, Ladley BA, eds. *Dental Instruments.* St. Louis: CV Mosby Co, 1981.

Chasteen JE. *Essentials of Clinical Dentistry Assisting,* 4th ed. St. Louis: CV Mosby Co, 1989.

Chen PS. *Chemistry: Inorganic, Organic and Biological,* 2nd ed. New York: Harper & Row Publisher Inc, 1980.

Christensen GJ. *Glass Ionomer as a Luting Material.* J Am Dent Assoc. 1990; 120: 55–57.

Ciancio SG, Bourgault PC. *Clinical Pharmacology for Dental Professionals,* 3rd ed. Chicago: Year Book Medical Publishers, Inc, 1989.

Cochran DL, Kalkwarf K, Brunsvold M. *Plaque and Calculus Removal Considerations for the Professional.* Chicago: Quintessence Publishing Co, Inc., 1994.

Cottone JA, Molinari JA, Terezhalmy G. *Practical Infection Control in Dentistry,* 2nd ed., Mavern, PA: Lea & Febiger, 1996.

Craig RG. *Restorative Dental Materials,* 9th ed. St. Louis: CV Mosby Co, 1993.

Davis K. *Training Manual for Oral and Maxillofacial Surgery Assistants,* 3rd ed. Lomita, CA: King Printing, 1996.

deLyre WR, Johnson N. *Essentials of Dental Radiology for Dental Assistants and Hygienists,* 5th ed. Stamford, CT: Appleton & Lange, 1995.

Domer LR, Snyder TL, Heid DW, eds. *Dental Practice Management.* St. Louis: CV Mosby Co, 1980.

Eastman Kodak Company. *Successful Panoramic Radiography.* Rochester, NY, 1993.

Eastman Kodak Company. *Quality Assurance in Dental Radiography.* Rochester, NY, 1990.

Eastman Kodak Company. *X-rays in Dentistry.* Rochester, NY, 1977.

Eastman Kodak Company. *Radiation Safety in Dental Radiography.* Rochester, NY, 1990.

Ehrlich A. *Business Administration for the Dental Assistant,* 4th ed., Colwell Systems, Champaign, IL, 1991.

Ehrlich A. *Nutrition and Dental Health.* Albany, NY: Delmar Publications, 1987.

*Facts About AIDS for the Dental Team,* 2nd ed. American Dental Association Council on Dental Therapeutics, Chicago: American Dental Association, October 1988.

Finkbeiner BL, Johnson CS. *Comprehensive Dental Assisting,* St. Louis: CV Mosby, 1994.

Finkbeiner BL, Patt JC. *Practice Management for the Dental Team,* 3rd ed., St. Louis: CV Mosby, 1991.

Frommer HH. *Radiology for Dental Auxiliaries,* 5th ed. St. Louis: CV Mosby Co, 1992.

Fuller JL, Denehy GE. *Concise Dental Anatomy and Morphology,* 2nd ed. Chicago: Year Book Medical Publishers, Inc, 1984.

Gilmore HW, et al. *Operative Dentistry,* 4th ed. St. Louis: CV Mosby Co, 1982.

Giunta JL. *Oral Pathology,* 3rd ed. Philadelphia: BC Decker, Inc, 1989.

Goss CM. *Gray's Anatomy,* 30th ed. Philadelphia: Lea & Febiger Publishers, 1985.

Goth A. *Medical Pharmacology,* 10th ed. St. Louis: CV Mosby Co, 1981.

Guthrie HA. *Human Nutrition,* St. Louis: CV Mosby Co, 1994.

Harris NO, Christen AG. *Primary Preventive Dentistry,* 4th ed. Stamford, CT: Appleton & Lange, 1994.

Hefferson JJ, Ayer WA, Koehler HM, eds. Foods, *Nutrition and Dental Health.* Volume I. South, IL: Pathodox Publishers, 1980.

Hooley J, Whitacre R. *Medications Used in Oral Surgery,* 3rd ed. Seattle: Stoma Press, Inc, 1984.

*Infection Control in the Dental Environment.* Department of Veterans Affairs, American Dental Association, Department of Health and Human Services and Centers for Disease Control. Washington DC: Eastern Dental Education Center Learning Resources Center Veterans Administration, 1989.

Jawetz E, et al. *Review of Medical Microbiology,* 20th ed. Stamford, CT: Appleton & Lange, 1995.

Keeton WT. *Biological Science,* 3rd ed. New York: WW Norton and Co, 1980.

Kumar, Angell M. *Basic Pathology,* 5th ed. Philadelphia: WB Saunders Co, 1992.

Ladley BA, Wilson SA. *Review of Dental Assisting.* St. Louis: CV Mosby Co, 1980.

Langland OE. *Radiography for Dental Hygienists & Dental Assistants,* 3rd ed. Springfield, IL: Charles C Thomas Publishers, 1988.

Little JW, Falace DA. *Dental Management of the Medically Compromised Patient,* 4th ed. St. Louis: CV Mosby, 1993.

Malamed SF. *Handbook of Medical Emergencies in the Dental Office,* 4th ed. St. Louis: CV Mosby Co, 1993.

Manson-Hing LR. *Fundamentals of Dental Radiography,* 3rd ed. Philadelphia: Lea & Febiger Publishers, 1990.

Miles D, Van Dis M, Jensen C, Ferretti A. *Radiographic Imaging for Dental Auxiliaries,* 2nd ed., Philadelphia: WB Saunders, 1993.

Miller CH, Palenik CJ. *Infection Control and Management of Hazardous Materials for the Dental Team.* St. Louis: CV Mosby Co, 1994.

Miller BF, Keane CB. *Encyclopedia and Dictionary of Medicine, Nursing, and Allied Health,* 4th ed. Philadelphia: WB Saunders Co, 1987.

Miller F. *College Physics,* 6th ed. New York: Harcourt Brace Jovanovich, Inc, 1987.

Muma RD, Lyons B, Borucki MJ, Pollard RB. *HIV Manual for Health Care Professionals.* Stamford, CT: Appleton & Lange, 1994.

Newman HN. *Dental Plaque.* Springfield, IL: Charles C Thomas Publishers, 1980.

Olson S. *Dental Radiography Laboratory Manual.* Philadelphia: WB Saunders Co, 1995.

Orban B. *Oral Histology and Embryology,* 9th ed. St. Louis: CV Mosby Co, 1980.

Peterson LJ. *Contemporary Oral and Maxillofacial Surgery,* 2nd ed. St. Louis: CV Mosby Co, 1993.

Philips RN. *Elements of Dental Materials for Dental Hygienists and Assistants,* 5th ed. Philadelphia: WB Saunders Co, 1994.

Randolph PM, Dennison CI. *Diet, Nutrition, and Dentistry.* St. Louis: CV Mosby Co, 1981.

Richardson RE, Barton RE. *The Dental Assistant,* 6th ed. New York: McGraw-Hill Inc, 1988.

Rose LF, Kaye D. *Internal Medicine For Dentistry,* 2nd ed. St. Louis: CV Mosby Co, 1990.

Rowe AHR, Alexander AG. *Clinical Methods, Medicine, Pathology and Pharmacology—A Companion to Dental Studies,* Vol 2. Boston: Blackwell Scientific Publications, 1988.

Sande MA, Volberding PA. *The Medical Management of AIDS,* 4th ed. Philadelphia: WB Saunders Co, 1994.

Schwarzrock SP, Jensen JR. *Effective Dental Assisting,* 7th ed. Dubuque, IA: William C Brown Co, 1991.

*Section on Instructional System Design,* Department of Pediodontology, School of Dentistry, University of California, San Francisco. Plaque Control Instruction. Berkley, CA: Praxis Publishing Co, 1978.

Seymour RA, Walton JG. *Adverse Drug Reactions in Dentistry.* New York: Oxford University Press, 1989.

Shafer WG, Hine MK, Levy BM. *Textbook of Oral Pathology,* 4th ed. Philadelphia: WB Saunders Co, 1983.

Shin D, Avers J. *AIDS/HIV Reference Guide for Medical Professionals.* West Los Angeles, CA: CIRID/UCLA School of Medicine, Publishers, 1988.

Sicher H. *Sicher's Oral Anatomy,* 8th ed. St. Louis: CV Mosby Co, 1988.

Skinner EW, Philips RW. *Skinner's Science of Dental Materials,* 9th ed. Philadelphia: WB Saunders Co, 1991.

Smith DC. *Dental Cements.* Adv Dent Res. 1988; 2:134–141.

Spohn EE, Halouski WA, Berry TC. *Operative Dentistry Procedures for Dental Auxiliaries.* St. Louis: CV Mosby Co, 1981.

*Supplement—Handling Hazardous Chemicals General Guidelines,* American Dental Association, 1995.

Suzuki M, Jordan R. *Glass Ionomer—Composite Sandwich Technique. J. Am Dent Assoc. 1990; 120: 55–57.*

Thibodeau GA. *Anatomy and Physiology,* 3rd ed. St. Louis: CV Mosby Co, 1995.

Torres H, Ehrlich A, Bird D, Dietz E. *Modern Dental Assisting,* 5th ed. Philadelphia: WB Saunders Co, 1995.

Tyldesley WR. *Oral Medicine,* 3rd ed. New York: Oxford University Press, 1990.

U.S. Department of Labor, Office of Health Compliance Assistance. OSHA Hazard Communication Standard, *Code of Federal Regulations, #29,* Part 1910 et al, February 9, 1994.

U.S. Department of Labor, Occupational Safety and Health Administration. *Controlling Occupational Exposure to Bloodborne Pathogens in Dentistry.* OSHA Publication 3129, 1992.

U.S. Department of Labor, Occupational Safety and Health Administration. *Chemical Hazard Communication.* OSHA Publication 3084 (Revised), 1988.

U.S. Department of Labor, Occupational Safety and Health Administration. *Hazard Communication Guidelines for Compliance.* OSHA Publication 3111, 1988.

Veterans Administration Medical Center. *Periodontal Resident Manual.* West Los Angeles: VA Medical Center, 1990.

Wheeler S. *An Atlas of Tooth Form,* 5th ed. Philadelphia: WB Saunders Co, 1984.

Wheeler S. *Dental Anatomy, Physiology and Occlusion,* 7th ed. Philadelphia: WB Saunders Co, 1992.

Wilkins EM. *Clinical Practice of the Dental Hygienist,* 7th ed. Philadelphia: Lea & Febiger, 1994.

Woodall IR. *Legal, Ethical, and Management Aspects of the Dental Care System,* 3rd ed. St. Louis: CV Mosby Co, 1987.

Wuehrmann A, Manson-Hing LR. *Dental Radiology,* 5th ed. St. Louis: CV Mosby Co, 1981.

Zwemer TJ. *Boucher's Clinical Dental Terminology,* 4th ed. St. Louis: CV Mosby Co, 1993.

# Index